Aids to Physiotherapy

Edited by
Jennifer M. Lee

BA MCSP DipTP
Principal of South Teesside School of Physiotherapy,
General Hospital, Middlesbrough

CHURCHILL LIVINGSTONE
EDINBURGH LONDON AND NEW YORK 1978

CHURCHILL LIVINGSTONE
Medical Division of Longman Group Limited

Distributed in the United States of America by
Longman Inc., 19 West 44th Street, New York,
N.Y. 10036 and by associated companies,
branches and representatives throughout the world.

ISBN 0 443 01581 3

British Library Cataloguing in Publication Data
Aids to physiotherapy.
  1. Pathology 2. Physical therapy
  I. Lee, Jennifer M
  616'.002'4616   RB111   78–40040

Printed in Singapore by
Singapore Offset Printing Pte Ltd

Aids to Physiotherapy

Preface

This book is intended to provide a concise aid to physiotherapy
students revising for their Part II examination. The contents of the book
are therefore limited to the Part II syllabus.

The book provides information in 'skeleton' form and students are
recommended to use the suggested bibliography to 'put the muscles
on' each clinical area. The early chapters are designed to refresh the
student's mind on *basic* professional skills and attitudes to patients, and
to assist the understanding of a patient's reactions, and those of his
family, to illness and disability. The later chapters on clinical conditions
are fact-packed lists of essential information on assessment, clinical
signs and symptoms and treatment.

I should like to thank the various contributors for their work in the
preparation of this book, also the publisher and the editor for their
forebearance and help.

1978   J.M.L.

Acknowledgements

Mr D. A. Hill would like to express thanks to Mrs P. McDowell for typing his contribution to the book. Mrs J. M. Abery wishes to express her grateful thanks to Dr A. G. Mowat, Consultant Rheumatologist at the Nuffield Orthopaedic Centre for advice with the text and for his help and encouragement. Miss J. A. Lamb expresses her thanks to Miss M. Rogers for typing her part of the manuscript. Miss K. J. Wallace would like to thank her colleagues for their help in the preparation of her section. Mr H. Standeven would like to thank Dr I. Adams and the staff of the Sports Clinic at St James' Hospital, Leeds for their co-operation and help with his section of the book. Miss B. M. Graveling would like to thank Mr A. Gibbs, Senior Orthopaedic Registrar, Norfolk and Norwich Hospital for reading the script, Mrs M. West for typing. Miss M. A. Auld thanks Dr A. Downey, Mr C. P. Blaikelock and Miss R. E. J. Lane for their help and advice with her part of the book. Mrs P. J. Foord would like to thank her husband, Dr K. D. Foord, whose help in the preparation and typing was invaluable. Miss J. M. Lee wishes to thank Mrs H. D. Simpson for typing her part of the script.

Contributors

Joan M. Abery, M.C.S.P., Senior Physiotherapist, Nuffield Orthopaedic Centre, Oxford.

Moira A. Auld, M.C.S.P., Superintendent Physiotherapist, Royal Infirmary, Aberdeen.

Paula J. Foord, M.C.S.P., Assistant Superintendent Physiotherapist, Nether Edge Hospital, Sheffield.

Beryl M. Graveling, M.C.S.P., Dip.T.P., District/Superintendent Physiotherapist, Norfolk and Norwich Hospital, Norwich.

David A. Hill, B.Sc., M.C.S.P., Dip.T.P., Reader, School of Health Sciences, Ulster College, Northern Ireland Polytechnic, Newtonabbey, Northern Ireland.

Julia A. Lamb, F.C.S.P., Dip.T.P., Senior Teacher, Wolverhampton School of Physiotherapy, Wolverhampton.

Jennifer M. Lee, B.A., M.C.S.P., Dip.T.P., Principal, South Teeside School of Physiotherapy, Ayresome Green Lane, Middlesbrough, Cleveland.

Harvey Standeven, M.C.S.P., Dip.T.P., Teacher, School of Physiotherapy, Leeds.

K. Julie Wallace, M.C.S.P., Senior Physiotherapist, The Jessop Hospital for Women, Sheffield.

Contributors

Contents

Contents

Movement

CLINICAL ASSESSMENT OF JOINT MOVEMENT

Classification of joints:
1. FIBROUS
   - (i) Bony surfaces joined by fibrous tissue
   - (ii) Little appreciable movement
   - (iii) Types e.g. suture, gomphosis and syndesmosis
2. CARTILAGINOUS
   - (i) Bony surfaces joined by cartilage
   - (ii) Limited movement
   - (iii) Types e.g. synchondrosis and symphysis
3. SYNOVIAL
   - (i) Bony surfaces not joined
   - (ii) Bony surfaces covered with hyaline cartilage
   - (iii) Joint cavity
   - (iv) Articular capsule
   - (v) Synovial membrane
   - (vi) Synovial fluid
   - (vii) Ligaments
   - (viii) Variety of movements possible
   - (ix) Types include ball and socket, condylar, plane, hinge, ellipsoid, saddle and pivot

Normal limiting factors to movement:
1. Ligaments
2. Joint surfaces
3. Muscles
4. Connective tissue
5. Other parts of body

Reasons for limitation of movement:
1. Destruction of intra-articular structures
2. Displacement of intra-articular body
3. Muscle disorder e.g. spasm, spasticity, weakness, flaccidity
4. Superficial scar tissue
5. Extra-articular and muscle adhesions

Measurement of joint movement:
1. Goniometer
2. Tracings
3. Ruler/tape measure
4. Mathematical determination
5. X-Rays/photographs

Recording Methods:
1. Numerical recording
2. Joint diagrams
3. Cumulative measurements plotted on graph
4. X-Rays/photographs

Principles of assessment of joint movement:
1. Patient's notes
2. Symptomatic enquiry
3. Position patient with joint uncovered
4. Fixation of adjacent joints
5. Observe joint for, posture, swelling, redness, muscle appearance, scars, skin colour and texture
6. Palpate for joint temperature, type and amount swelling, tenderness, normal shape of joint
7. Check movement:
    (i) Actively for ability to do voluntary movement, limitation of movement, pain, co-ordination, trick movements, muscle weakness or spasm, skin contractions
    (ii) Passively for ease of movement, limitation, muscle weakness/spasm, pain, crepitus
    (iii) Resisted movement for power through range and pain
8. Function
    (i) Lower limb joints check gait, stairs, turning
    (ii) Upper limb joints check hand function
    (iii) Trunk joints check transfers
9. Check general posture
10. Record findings
11. Reassess periodically e.g. fortnightly intervals

Mobilization of joint movement

Local relaxation:
1. Contrast method
2. Reciprocal method
3. Pendular movement
4. Rhythmical passive movements
5. Neuromuscular facilitation e.g. hold-relax, contract-relax, Bobath
6. Massage
7. Hydrotherapy

Passive movement:
1. Relaxed
2. Forced
3. Stretch single and multi-joint muscles
4. Maitland mobilizations
5. Auto-assisted pulley circuits

Active assisted movement:
1. Pendular exercises
2. Suspension
3. Hydrotherapy
4. Neuromuscular facilitation

Free active movement:
1. Eccentric and concentric muscle work through full range
2. Use of lever length of limb
3. Variations in starting position
4. Speed
5. Duration of exercise

To support functional range:
1. Splints — Serial, 'lively', supporting, collars, corsets

Electrical techniques used to improve joint movement:
1. Heat — IRR, paraffin wax, hot packs, microwave, SWD
2. Ultrasound
3. Faradism

CLINICAL ASSESSMENT OF MUSCLE FUNCTION
1. Isotonic − concentric, eccentric
2. Isometric/Static

Range of muscle work:
1. Outer − full stretch to mid-point contraction
2. Inner − mid-point to full contraction
3. Middle − middle outer to middle inner range

Group action of muscles:
1. Agonists/Prime Movers − produce required movement
2. Antagonists − controlled relaxation to allow movement
3. Synergists − assist action of agonists
4. Fixators − stabilize attachments of agonists, antagonists and synergists

Cause of muscle weakness:
1. Intrinsic muscle disease
2. Lower motor neurone lesion
3. Lesions AHC
4. Lesions of upper motor neurone
5. Disordered proprioceptive input
6. Ischaemia
7. Disuse atrophy
8. Joint disease
9. Psychological

Measurement of muscle function:
1. Oxford scale
   0 − Nil contraction
   1 − Flicker contraction
   2 − Contraction if gravity counterbalanced
   3 − Contraction against gravity only
   4 − Contraction against gravity and weight
   5 − Normal function
2. Manual Muscle Examination Record using good, poor, nil to assess contraction
3. 1. Repetition maximum
4. Tensiometer

Recording methods:
1. Numerical
2. Cumulative muscle chart

Principles of assessment of muscle function:
1. Read patient's notes
2. Symptomatic enquiry
3. Patient positioned and adequately undressed
4. Observation and measurement of muscle bulk
5. Comparison with 'normal' side
6. Assess muscle function i.e. Oxford scale in all ranges/subjective assessment of endurance
7. Check for pain on contraction
8. Identify spasm/spasticity/rigidity/flaccidity
9. Assess functional use of affected limb/trunk
10. Record findings
11. Reassess at weekly intervals

Prevention of muscle atrophy:
1. Isometric exercises – for painful/immobilized joints
2. Isotonic exercises – for pain free and mobile joints
3. PNF – facilitate contraction
4. Passive movements – maintain proprioceptive input to AHC and cortex
5. Electrical procedures – faradism to initiate contraction: IDC to maintain muscle properties

Re-education of muscle:
1. Hypotonicity – flaccidity
2. Hypertonicity – spasticity, spasm, rigidity
3. Strengthening
4. Endurance
5. Co-ordination of muscle activity
   1. Hypotonicity
     Techniques for facilitating muscle contraction:
      (i)   Fast brusning
      (ii) Facilitatory icing   ⎱ Individually or in combination to
      (iii) Vibration   ⎰ appropriate dermatome/muscle
      (iv) Slapping   belly/tendon
      (v)   Use of visual/auditory stimuli
      (vi) PNF – successive induction
      (vii) Righting and equilibrium reactions
      (viii) Irradiation from movement of strong muscle groups
      (ix) Longitudinal compression
      (x)   Longitudinal 'pounding'
      (xi) Other Rood techniques

2. Hypertonicity
   (i) To reduce spasticity:
        Positioning
        a. Bobath inhibitory position
        b. Shaking
        Movement
        a. Reciprocal relaxation
        b. PNF techniques e.g. hold – relax, slow reversals
        Passive movements – rhythmical
        Ice Pack – (20–30 min)
        Immersion in cold water (10 min)
        Relaxation – general
        Massage – rhythmical, deep kneading
        Heat – variable in effect
   (ii) Spasm – primary aim is to reduce pain and thereby
        spasm by:
        a. Application of heat e.g. hot pack, IRR, SWD,
            microwave, US
        b. Application of cold e.g. ice pack, immersion,
            ice cube massage
        c. Ethyl chloride spray
        d. Relaxation techniques
        e. Passive movement
        f. Maitland mobilizations
        g. Hydrotherapy
        h. Active assisted exercises e.g. pendular
        i. Free active exercises.
        j. PNF e.g. hold – relax/contract – relax, slow
            reversals
   (iii) Rigidity:
        a. Passive movements 'pumping up'
        b. Trunk rotation – limb rotation
        c. Use righting responses to gain movement
        d. Transfers
        e. Free active movement – facilitation of
            movement patterns

3. Increase muscle power
    (i)   Isometric exercises
    (ii)   Isotonic exercises: type muscle work speed, lever length
    (iii)   Manual resistance
    (iv)   PNF
    (v)   Progressive resistance exercises e.g. de Lorme
    (vi)   Brief maximal exercises
    (vii)   Use of body weight
    (viii) Springs/weights
    (ix)   Maleable resistances
    (x)   Underwater resistance
    (xi)   Static machines e.g. rowing machine
4. Increase muscle endurance
    (i)   Isotonic exercises
    (ii)   Progressive resistance exercises e.g. McQueen
    (iii)   Use of body weight
    (iv)   Springs
    (v)   Static bicycle/rowing machine
    (vi)   Endurance gym circuit
5. Co-ordination of muscle activity
    (i)   Mat exercises — transfers and stabilization
    (ii)   Lateral trunk/girdle movements
    (iii)   Joint approximation
    (iv)   PNF to limbs e.g. holds in range, slow reversals
    (v)   Progression of starting positions
    (vi)   Balance and righting reflexes
    (vii)   Weight resisted exercises
    (viii) Frenkels
    (ix)   Functional activities

Co-ordination and balance

Control
1. Sensory input
   (i)   Cutaneous
   (ii) Proprioceptive
   (iii) Special senses
2. Central co-ordination
   (i)   Cerebrum and basal ganglia
   (ii) Brain stem nuclei
   (iii) Cerebellum
3. Effector system
   (i)   Upper motor neurone pathways
   (ii) Lower motor neurone pathways

Causes of inco-ordination
1. Weak muscle groups
2. Pain/spasm
3. Spasticity
4. Loss sensory input
5. Spinal cord lesion
6. Cerebellar lesion
7. Brain stem/basal ganglia lesion

Principles of treatment
1. Correct imbalance of muscle power
2. Relieve pain
3. Reduce spasticity
4. Inhibit formation or increase of spasticity
Use other intact senses to gain feed-back on body position

Methods
1. PNF – rhythmic stabilizations, slow reversals
2. Approximation of joints
3. Progression of starting position
4. Balance and righting reflexes
5. Frenkels exercises
6. Functional activities

Re-education of gait

Assessment:
1. Read patient's notes
2. Assess joint range and muscle power in lower limb
3. Analyse gait (if possible)
4. Assess walking aid requirements
5. Assess muscle power in upper limbs

Preparation for walking
Aims to:
1. Strengthen extensor mechanism of upper limbs
2. Improve balance in sitting
3. Gain trunk mobility
4. Strengthen weight bearing limb
5. Teach hip hitching and active exercises to non-weight bearing limb
6. Ensure walking aid is correct size for patient
7. Demonstrate gait to patient
8. Teach sitting to standing and reverse
9. Teach gait

Methods of walking with aids
1. Non weight bearing
2. Partial weight bearing
3. Full weight bearing

Types of aid
1. Crutches — axillary, elbow or gutter
2. Tripods/quadropods
3. Frame — fixed or reciprocal
4. Sticks

Aims of re-education of walking
1. To improve balance in standing
2. To teach, turns, stairs, side-step and reverse steps
3. To progress gait pattern
4. To reduce support of aid
5. To analyse and correct gait faults

Some gait faults
1. Uneven step timing
2. Unequal length stride
3. Incorrect weight distribution on each foot
4. Abduction gait
5. Incorrect weight transference through weight bearing foot

Re-education of posture

Cause poor posture
1. Structural abnormalities
2. Muscle imbalance
3. Pain/tension
4. Neurological disorders
5. Debilitating disease
6. Occupational strains
7. Psychological

Assessment of posture
1. Patient's medical history
2. Observe static posture
   (i)   from front, side, back
   (ii) Measure limb length
   (iii) Measure joint range
   (iv) Measure muscle strength
3. Observe dynamic posture
   (i)   Trunk movements
   (ii) Feeding/dressing patterns
   (iii) Walking
4. Check for pain/spasm on movement
5. Test tendon reflexes
6. Record findings

Principles of treatment
1. Relieve pain
2. Gain relaxation of area
3. Mobilize affected joints
4. Strengthen weak muscles
5. Correct faulty muscle mechanics
6. Teach normal postural patterns by 'feel' and vision
7. Assess for supportive or corrective devices
8. Advice on home/occupational work postures

Methods
1. Heat e.g. IRR, SWD, microwave
2. Hydrotherapy/suspension
3. Active assisted/free active movements
4. Isometric exercises
5. Isotonic exercises
6. Manual, spring or weight resistance
7. Facilitation techniques
8. Teach back and neck care
9. Re-educate gait
10. Functional ADL activities

Re-education of respiratory movement

Cause of respiratory embarrassment
1. Respiratory and cardiac diseases
2. Structural disorders of thorax and vertebral column
3. Joint disease
4. Vascular disease
5. Post-operative lung infections

Assessment of respiratory movements
1. Read medical notes
2. Check posture and shape of chest
3. Assess chest expansion
4. Vitalograph readings
5. Cough and sputum
6. Range of movement thoracic spine and shoulder girdle and joint
7. Exercise tolerance
See also pp. 72 and 84

Principles of treatment to:
1. Maintain clear airway
2. Teach correct breathing pattern
3. Remove secretions
4. Teach coughing
5. Improve movement in thorax, spine and shoulder girdle
6. Improve exercise tolerance

Methods
1. Relaxation general/local
2. Breathing exercises – general and local
3. Varying starting positions
4. Postural drainage
5. Cough-belt
6. Vibrations, shaking, percussion
7. General exercises, and posture correction
8. IPPB
See section on Cardio-respiratory disease

Hydrotherapy

Physiological effects
1. Rise in body temperature
2. Increased sweating
3. Superficial vasodilitation
4. Increase in peripheral circulation
5. Heart and respiratory rates increased
6. Blood pressure falls after immersion
7. Increased metabolism
8. Sedative effect on sensory nerve endings
9. Relaxation of muscle
10. Easily fatigued

Used to:
1. Induce muscle relaxation
2. Relieve pain
3. Mobilize joints
4. Assist weak muscles to contract
5. Resist muscle work
6. Allows non weight bearing walking
7. Encourage recreational activities
8. Achieve psychological effect

Disadvantages
1. Individual's fear of water
2. Rapid fatigue
3. Danger of infection
4. Difficult to fix joints and isolate movement

Procedure prior to entering pool
1. Read patient's notes
2. Check skin and continence
3. Assess mobility and strength
4. Explain treatment
5. Assess attitude to treatment
6. Patient takes shower
7. Enters antiseptic foot bath
8. Enters pool

Procedure after treatment
1. Shower
2. Pack in absorbent sheet and blanket
3. Bed rest for 20–30 min
4. Give drink
5. Dress
6. Allow further cooling off period prior to leaving building

Dosage, start 5 min–30 min

Contraindications
1. Skin infection or lesions
2. Cardiovascular disorders
3. Respiratory distress

Technical notes
1. Water temperature 34°–37°C
2. Water changed every 4 hours
3. Chlorination 0.5–0.75 parts per million
4. pH 7.2–8.0
5. Test pH and chlorination twice daily
6. Check stretchers, hoists and equipment weekly
7. Antiseptic foot bath changed twice daily
8. Pool area temperature 23°–24°C
9. Changing area 18°–19°C
10. Humidity 50–60 per cent

Relaxation
Definition: muscles free from abnormal tension

Causes of muscle tension
1. Disorders of CNS causing spasticity/rigidity
2. Pain causing spasm
3. State of mind

Methods of gaining relaxation of muscle
General relaxation
1. Well supported position
2. Quiet restful surroundings
3. Contrast method
4. Reciprocal method
Other techniques
5. Hydrotherapy
6. Total suspension
7. Cold immersion techniques

Local relaxation
1. Contrast method
2. Reciprocal method
3. Rhythmical passive movements
4. PNF e.g. hold – relax/contract – relax
5. Hydrotherapy
6. Local suspension
7. Free active pendular movements
8. Massage
9. Local heat e.g. hot packs, IRR, SWD, microwave
10. Local cold

Thermal, electrical and manipulative procedures

Physiological effects of local heat
1. Increased tissue metabolism, Van't Hoff's Law
2. Increased superficial blood flow
3. Sedative effect on sensory nerve endings
4. Relaxation of muscle tissue

More general effects
1. Fall in BP
2. Increase in heart and respiratory rate
3. Rise in 'core' temperature
4. Increased activity of sweat glands

Precautions for all heat treatments
1. Test integrity of skin thermal sensation
2. Check adequate circulation
3. Test understanding of patient
4. Read medical history
5. Warn patient re treatment

Dangers to Use
1. Burns
2. Scalds
3. Syncope
4. Earth shock

SHORT WAVE DIATHERMY (SWD)

Technical notes
1. SWD uses wavelengths of the electromagnetic spectrum
2. Frequency 27 mega cycles/second
3. Wavelength 11m
4. Depth of penetration – full body
5. Greatest heating in fat tissue
6. Heat produced in tissues by dipole rotation and molecular distortion/eddy currents
7. Applied using condenser field or cable technique
8. Condenser field produces electrostatic field
9. Cable produces electrostatic and magnetic field
10. Dosage:
    Chronic conditions
    (i)   Intensity, comfortable-warmth
    (ii) Duration, maximum rise in tissue temperature at 20 min
    (iii) Frequency, daily
    Acute conditions:
    (i)   Intensity, below sensation warmth
    (ii) Duration $2\frac{1}{2}$–10 min
    (iii) Frequency BD

Used to
1. Assist resolution of acute inflammation
2. Relieve pain
3. Increase vascularity
4. Induce muscle relaxation
5. Reduce viscosity of joint fluids and tissues

Contraindications
1. Large area loss of skin sensation
2. Venous thrombus
3. Arterial insufficiency
4. Haemorrhage
5. Metal in tissues
6. Pregnancy
7. Neoplasm
8. TB
9. Deep X-Ray therapy
10. Cardiac pacemakers
11. Some intrauterine devices

MICROWAVE

Technical notes
1. Microwave uses wavelengths of the electromagnetic spectrum
2. Frequency 2450 megacycles/second, wavelength 12.25 cm
3. Depth of penetration – 3 cm
4. Irradiates one surface of body
5. Greatest heating in vascular tissues cf. SWD
6. Heat produced in tissues by absorption of radiation and conduction in tissues
7. Eye protection for all treatments
8. Dosage up to 200 watts; 10–30 min, daily

Used to
1. Increase circulation
2. Raise threshold pain nerve endings
3. Reduce muscle spasm

Contraindications
1. Large area loss of thermal sensation
2. Not used near eyes, gonads, growing bone
3. Haemorrhage
4. Neoplasm and TB
5. Ischaemic conditions
6. Metal implants
7. Pregnancy
8. Severe oedema
9. Wet dressings

INFRA-RED RADIATION (IRR)

Technical notes
1. Non-luminous generator
2. Electromagnetic wavelength 4000–7700 Å
3. Shorter wavelengths produce greatest heating effect
4. Depth of penetration, 1–10 mm
5. Heat produced by absorption of radiant energy
6. Dosage 20–30 min, daily
7. IRR obey optical laws

Used to
1. Relieve pain
2. Relax superficial muscle spasm
3. Increase superficial blood-supply

Contraindications
1. Loss of large area of thermal skin sensation
2. Some skin diseases
3. Vascular insufficiency
4. Haemorrhage
5. Some skin liniments

ULTRA-SOUND (US)

Physiological effects
1. Thermal (unpulsed US)
   (i) Rise in tissue temperature, greatest in muscle
   (ii) Vasodilitation
2. Non Thermal (pulsed US)
   (i) Micromassage
   (ii) Analgesia

Technical notes
1. US is a form of acoustic vibration
2. Frequency 0.8–1 megacycle per second, wavelength 1.5 mm
3. Depth of penetration varies with frequency and nature of tissue
4. Half value distance e.g. 1 000 000 cycles/second, $\frac{1}{2}$ value
   at 5 cm
5. Pulsed beam produces mechanical effect
6. Unpulsed beam produces thermal and mechanical effects
7. Dosage – acute conditions – 0.25–1.0 w/cm² BD 3 min
   chronic conditions – 1.0–3.0 w/cm² alt. days 8–10 min
   Depends on depth structure $\frac{1}{2}$ value distance
8. Application, either contact or immersion
9. Coupling medium usually necessary stationary/moving head
   technique

Used to
1. Remove oedema
2. Increase blood supply
3. Reduce pain
4. Mobilize collagen tissues
5. Assist relaxation of muscle spasm

Contraindications
1. Care when treating areas adjacent to eyes, ear, testes and ovaries
2. Impaired circulation
3. Thrombus formation
4. Neoplasm and TB
5. Acute sepsis
6. DXRT and isotope treatment
7. Haemophiliacs

ULTRA-VIOLET RADIATION

Physiological effects
1. Four degrees erythema reaction (2500 Å and 3000 Å)
2. Epidermal thickening
3. Desquamation
4. Pigmentation (2300–3400 Å)
5. Abiotic effect (2500–2700 Å)
6. Formation Vitamin D (2800 Å)
7. Psychological effect

Technical notes
UVR part of
1. Electromagnetic spectrum 3900–1849 Å
2. Depth of penetration 1.5 mm
3. Application in contact, 18 in or 36 in
4. Filters to absorb different wavelengths
5. Dosage:
   skin test for E_1o; to repeat E_1o add 25 per cent previous dose
   E_2^o is $E_1^o \times 2\frac{1}{2}$; to repeat E_2^o add 50 per cent previous dose
   E_3^o is $E_1^o \times 5$; to repeat E_3^o add 75 per cent previous dose
   E_4^o is $E_1^o \times 10$; to repeat E_4^o add 100 per cent previous dose
   suberythermal dose $\frac{1}{2}-\frac{2}{3}$ of E_1^o
   To calculate dose at new distance.
   $$\text{New dose} = \frac{\text{Old dose} \times \text{new distance}^2}{\text{Old distance}^2}$$

Used to
1. Stimulate growth new skin
2. Produce pigmentation
3. Exfoliation
4. Improve superficial circulation
5. Heal wounds
6. Counter-irritant effect
7. Produce Vitamin D
8. Reduce infection
9. Psychological effect

Contraindications
1. Individual sensitivity
2. Sensitizing drugs e.g. some antibiotics, tranquillizers, steroids
3. Certain diseases e.g. TB, eczema
4. Deep X-Ray therapy

LOW FREQUENCY MUSCLE STIMULATING CURRENTS

Faradic type current

Physiological effects:
1. Stimulation sensory and motor nerve
2. Facilitate muscle contraction
3. Increase muscle metabolism
4. Vasodilitation of deep and superficial blood vessels
5. Increased arterial supply
6. 'Muscle-pump' action improves venous and lymphatic drainage

Used to
1. Re-educate muscle action
2. Train new muscle function
3. Increase circulation
4. Prevent/stretch adhesions
5. Hypertrophy muscle

Technical notes
1. Faradic type current is an alternating current
2. Pulse lengths 0.1–1.0 ms
3. Frequency 50–100 pulses per second
4. Surged
5. Dosage, cease when voluntary contraction achieved

Interrupted direct current

Physiological effects:
1. Stimulation of sensory nerves
2. Contracts denervated muscle
3. Increases blood supply
4. Improves venous and lymphatic drainage
5. Chemical effects

Used to
1. Maintain properties of muscle
2. Improve circulation
3. Test muscle for reinnervation (SDC)
4. Prevent contractures

Technical notes
1. Depolarized IDC
2. Pulse length between 300 ms–0.03 ms
3. Pulse shape: triangular, trapezoidal, saw tooth square wave
4. Frequency 30 impulses per min, can be varied
5. Dosage: minimum of 90 contractions per muscle per day

COLD THERAPY

Physiological effects of local cold

Effect on nerve tissue:
1. Brief cutaneous cooling 3–5 s increases input to CNS and enhances motor output
2. Longer period of cooling 5–7 min diminishes sensation
3. Prolonged period of cooling 20–30 min diminishes muscle tone and nerve conduction velocity

Effect on circulation
1. Vasoconstriction – initially on application
2. Vasodilitation later in cold application

Effect on tissues
1. Reduces metabolic rate
2. Increases joint viscosity
3. Increases muscle viscosity
4. Produces longer contraction and relaxation time in muscle

Precautions
1. Care in arteriosclerotic heart disease
2. Ischaemic tissue
3. Hypertension – with care
4. Psychological
5. No cold to cutaneous area of vagus nerve

Contraindications
1. Circulatory disorders
2. Coronary heart disease
3. External haemorrhage
4. Cold allergy
5. Cold aversion

Used to
1. Control oedema formation and haemorrhage
2. Relieve pain
3. Reduce muscle spasm
4. Reduce muscle spasticity
5. Improve nerve transmission
6. Increase visual acuity
7. Facilitate muscle contraction
8. Improve sustained muscle contraction

Methods of application
1. Cold pack
2. Cold immersion of limb or lower trunk
3. Ice cube massage
4. Ethyl chloride spray
5. Contrast baths

MANIPULATIVE PROCEDURES

Terminology:

Effleurage   — stroking, gliding movements
Petrissage   — compression movements
Friction   — deep local massage
Vibration   — oscillatory to-and-fro movements
Percussion   — clapping
Tapotement   — percussion

EFFLEURAGE

Effleurage
1. Rhythmical
2. Deep/superficial centripetal gliding movements
3. One/two handed

Effects
1. Increases superficial lymphatic and venous flow
2. Mobilization of superficial soft tissues
3. Stimulates 'axon reflex'

Used to
1. Remove oedema
2. Stretch scar tissue
3. Relax muscles

Stroking
1. Rhythmical, superficial/deep movements
2. Speed variable
3. One or two handed

Effects
1. Sedative or stimulating to nervous system
2. Brisk stroking produces superficial vasodilitation

Used to
1. Relieve local muscle spasm
2. General relaxation
3. Stimulate superficial vasodilitation

PETRISSAGE

Kneading
1. Using palm/finger(s)
2. Depth and speed variable
3. One or two handed

Picking up
1. Lifting and squeezing muscle
2. One/two handed

Wringing
1. Lifting, squeezing wringing action of superficial soft tissues
2. Two handed

Skin rolling
1. Skin and subcutaneous tissues grasped and rolled between fingers
2. Two handed

Effects
1. Increase venous and lymphatic return
2. Superficial vasodilitation
3. Reduce muscle tone
4. Mobilize skin and fibrous tissue

Used to
1. Increase circulation
2. Sedative effect
3. Reduce spasm/spasticity
4. Mobilize scar tissue and adhesions

FRICTIONS

1. Circular/transverse movements
2. Using fingers of one/two hands
3. Pressure increases with application

Effects
1. Mobilize deep structures
2. Increases blood supply
3. Produces temporary analgesia
4. Reduces haematoma formation

Used to
1. Mobilize ligaments, tendons or tendon sheaths
2. Reduce haematoma

VIBRATION

Shaking
1. Rhythmic large amplitude shaking movement
2. One/two handed

Vibration
1. Rhythmic small amplitude movement
2. Constant manual pressure
3. One/two handed

Effects
To produce movement of gases and liquids

Used to
1. Remove secretions in lung
2. Reduce tissue effusion

TAPOTEMENT

Clapping
1. Relaxed, cupped hand
2. Alternate movement of hands

Effects
1. Mobilize secretions
2. Produces skin erythema

Used to
1. Remove bronchial secretions
2. Induce coughing
NB can increase pleural effusion

FURTHER READING

Duffield, M. H. ed. (1976) *Exercises in Water*. London: Bailliere.
Hollis, M. (1976) *Practical Exercise Therapy*. Oxford: Blackwell.
Lee, J. M. Warren, M. P. (1978) *Cold Therapy in Rehabilitation*.
    London: Bell & Hyman.
Licht, D. ed. (1960) *Massage Manipulation and Traction*. New Haven:
    Licht.
Licht, S. ed. (1963) *Medical Hydrology*. New Haven: Licht.
Licht, S. ed. (1965) *Therapeutic Exercises*. New Haven: Licht.
Licht, S. ed. (1965) *Therapeutic Exercises*. New Haven: Licht.
Licht, S. ed. (1967) *Therapeutic Electricity and Ultra Violet Radiation*.
    New Haven: Licht.
O'Connell A. L. & Gardner, E. B. (1972) *Understanding the Scientific
    Bases of Human Movement*. Baltimore: Williams and Wilkins.
Scott, P. (1975) *Claytons Electrotherapy and Actinotherapy*. London:
    Bailliere.
Summer, W. & Patrick, M. K. (1964) *Ultrasonic Therapy*. Amsterdam:
    Elsevier.

Behavioural sciences

Behavioural Science is the scientific study of behaviour and experience.
Behaviour can be objectively observed and recorded. Experience is
personal and subjective.

SCOPE OF BEHAVIOURAL SCIENCE

Considerable overlap exists between the following areas:
1. Developmental Psychology
2. Comparative Psychology
3. Physiological Psychology
4. Educational Psychology
5. Organizational Psychology
6. Clinical Psychology
7. Social Psychology
8. Sociology

Different schools of psychology may appear to be contradictory, but are
better regarded as complementary.
Behaviourists claim to be interested only in behaviour.
Cognitive schools study conscious awareness.

DEVELOPMENTAL PSYCHOLOGY

Aspects
1. Physical development and growth (dealt with in Anatomy and Physiology)
2. Mental and perceptual development
3. Moral development

Stages of Mental and Perceptual Development (Piaget)
(i) Sensory motor stage — Birth to Eighteen months.
Child is born with certain reflexes e.g. sucking, grasping. These reflexes are rapidly adapted into more purposeful movements in response to specific stimuli. There is little evidence of imagery, or mental representation of objects in the outside world.
(ii) Pre-operational stage — Eighteen months to seven years.
Simple rules of arithmetic can be learned, but their implications are not fully mentally internalized. The child is therefore unable to appreciate conservation of physical properties of volume, mass or number. Perceptions are always from child's point of view i.e. ego-centric.
(iii) Concrete operational stage — Seven to eleven years.
Child now appreciates conservation of volume, mass and number. Perception shows awareness of relationships between separate objects and concepts.
(iv) Formal operational stage — Eleven years onwards.
Child is able to appreciate abstract concepts concerning behaviour of objects in the physical world e.g. buoyancy, momentum, velocity. Also able to appreciate and formulate universal rules and scientific laws involved with such concepts.

Moral development
Up to the age of six years children tend to judge good behaviour as that which is rewarded, and bad behaviour as that which is punished. Judgement is based on the consequences of the behaviour. By the age of ten intentionality plays a more important role in judging moral behaviour. During adolescence strong attitudes concerning clusters of political or religious values may develop, but their intensity usually mellows with age.

Learning–A change in behaviour as the result of experience.

Types of learning   Imprinting

Associative learning
{
Classical conditioning
Operant conditioning
Avoidance conditioning
Habituation learning
}

Latent Learning

Cognitive learning
{
Imitation
Insight
Creativity
}

Imprinting is the tendency of the newborn to follow the first moving object it sees, which in natural conditions is the mother. It occurs particularly in species which are mobile from birth e.g. chickens, cattle. There is some doubt as to whether it occurs in humans.

Classical conditioning occurs when the autonomic nervous system responds to a previously neutral stimulus. The stimulus has to be associated with another stimulus to which the autonomic system already responds. For example, pain causes specific responses.

If the therapist causes pain, then the sight or thought of the therapist may be sufficient to evoke the autonomic responses to pain. Some attitudes are formed as a result of classical conditioning.

Operant conditioning occurs when the voluntary muscles are used in order to obtain a reward. The reward reinforces the behaviour, and makes its repetition more likely. For example, if a patient feels better after attending for treatment, he is more likely to attend in future.

Avoidance conditioning occurs when an individual learns to behave in such a manner that he avoids unpleasant stimuli. Punishment may be used as an avoidance conditioner, and may take various forms e.g. physical, verbal.

Using bio-feedback techniques, operant conditioning of the autonomic nervous system is now possible. Some medical implications are:
(i)   Voluntary regulation of blood pressure
(ii)   Voluntary regulation of local body temperature (useful for migraine patients)
(iii) Voluntary regulation of EEG waves, which may be used to abort epileptic attacks

Habituation learning is a decreased response to repetitions of the same stimulus.
e.g. Patients anxiety responses may reduce with repeated visits for treatment.

Latent learning occurs in the apparent absence of either pleasant or unpleasant stimuli. Only neutral stimuli are present. Latent learning possibly satisfies a curiosity drive. Latent learning may prove useful at a later date.

Imitation learning occurs when the learner observes another's behaviour, and then matches their own behaviour to that of the observed model. This is formally used in demonstrations to students, patients etc.

Insight learning is problem solving. The individual draws on past experience to arrive at a solution which often occurs in 'a flash of inspiration'.

Creativity is the production of a completely new set of ideas. Inventiveness, or originality of thought in art, science, music etc.

Motor skill The learned ability to bring about predetermined results with maximum certainty, often with the minimum outlay of time or energy or both. (Guthrie)

Most physiotherapy treatments involve the teaching of motor skills to patients. Maturational skills e.g. walking rely on correct neurological development.

Reasons for practice of a skill
1. To acquire a new skill
2. To improve an existing skill
3. To maintain a high level of skill

Guidance of a skill can
1. Reduce the errors during practice
2. Shorten the time necessary to acquire skill
3. Result in a higher ultimate level of skill

Types of guidance
1. Verbal (explanation)
2. Visual (demonstration)
3. Manual (assisted or resisted)
4. Mechanical (assisted or resisted)

All types of guidance are relevant to physiotherapists especially during muscle training or re-education

Massed or spaced practice
In massed practice the skill is practised frequently with only short intervals between practice sessions. In spaced practice the intervals between sessions are longer

Optimum spacing varies with the complexity of the skill and the personality of the learner. Complex skills benefit from greater spacing.

Whole or part practice
The size or complexity of a skill will affect the optimum size of any part of the skill which can be learnt at one practice session e.g. The skill of manipulative treatments could not all be taught at one time. Optimum size of part will also be affected by the capacity of the learner, and should be considered for each patient learning or re-learning a skill.

Knowledge of results (feedback)
The learner acquires skill more rapidly if he is well informed concerning progress e.g. verbal reinforcement.

'Transfer' occurs when the learning of one skill affects the learning of another skill. Positive transfer facilitates learning between skills, and should be encouraged. Positive transfer occurs when the learning situations and skill requirements are similar e.g. Practising walking on a smooth gymnasium floor may not show much positive transfer if the patient has to walk across a ploughed field to get home.

Intelligence is the level of adaptability to environmental requirements.
Measurement
Intelligence Quotient (IQ) is an attempt to assign a numerical value to intelligent behaviour, based on comparing mental age with chronological age, up to the age of sixteen.

$$IQ = \frac{\text{Mental age}}{\text{Chronological age}} \times \frac{1}{100}$$

The concept of IQ is carried on into adult life.

For any individual, intelligence levels tend to be general across wide areas of intellectual ability, but some variation does exist in different aspects of intelligence. Some people may score high on verbal and educational factors, while others may score high on mechanical and mathematical factors.

Evidence suggests that intelligence is mainly heredity, but can be influenced by extremes of environment.

Perception is the organism's interpretation of internal and external environmental stimuli.

Some perceptual abilities are either innate, or rapidly learned by the newborn infant e.g. perception of a human face.

Other perceptual abilities are greatly modified by environment and experience, especially during development e.g. perception of distances or angles.

Perceptual constancy. People tend to perceive what they expect to perceive e.g. oval coins tend to be perceived as round. Pictures of grass tend to be perceived as green, even if the grass is another colour.

Perceptual defence. People tend to perceive what they want to perceive and may fail to perceive what they do not wish to perceive. For example, patients may refuse to perceive the truth concerning their illness or injury.

Memory is a mental reconstruction of past events. Short term memory is for immediate use e.g. looking at a phone number, then dialling it. Long term memory is a store of information, and can be improved by associative memories. (See associative learning) Time is required for the neurological changes resulting in consolidation of memory.

Consolidation may be prevented by concussion, resulting in retrograde amnesia, which is loss of memory backwards in time from the time of injury. Mental deterioration and ageing can also result in retrograde amnesia.

Personality is made up of a collection of behaviour tendencies (traits) of varying degrees e.g. aggression, generosity, ambition.

Two main dimensions are recognized.

1. Extraversion   —   Introversion
(likes constant   (likes quiet
excitement)   life)

Evidence suggests that Introverts have a more active ascending reticular system.

2. Neuroticism   —   Stability

May be related to activity of the autonomic nervous system.

Various traits interact within individuals to give a variety of personality types.

Innate tendencies interact with the environment and experience to produce the personality.

Motivation or drive

Some motivation is physiological e.g. hunger, thirst and sex drives are essential for survival and perpetuation of the species. Drives also exist to seek comfort, security and freedom from pain. Man is a social animal and when the above drives are satisfied he usually seeks the company and respect of others. Still higher motivations are creative e.g. art, music, drama.

Motivations may change dramatically when a person is ill, in pain, or confined to hospital. Therapists can develop the skill to steer the patient's motivation towards rehabilitation and recovery.

Emotion is a subjective experience (feeling)
Emotions such as fear, rage, pleasure correlate highly with physiological states. Evidence suggests that emotions are largely due to activity in various regions of the brain, especially the mid brain and limbic system. The therapist should be aware that brain damage can result in behavioural aspects of emotion occurring, while the subjective feelings are absent.

Physiological changes are usually produced as a result of emotional experience, but some evidence suggests that production of the appropriate physiological changes can likewise cause some elements of the correlated emotion e.g. excitement causes release of adrenaline, and injection of adrenaline makes a person more excitable.

Social Psychology
Humans tend to congregate in groups.
Each group develops norms of behaviour in the way they respond to each other in matters relating to birth, marriage, death, earning a living, feeding and an almost infinite range of activities. Such groups are known as cultures.

Socialization is the process by which the developing child is persuaded to conform to cultural norms by use of rewards (operant conditioning), punishments (avoidance conditioning) and imitation.

Adults who deviate widely from cultural norms usually find that the group exerts sanctions on them in an attempt to persuade them to return to the norm. Continual refusal to respond to such sanctions frequently results in a group decision to ignore the deviant.

Most people like to belong to, and be accepted and respected by a group. Some members emerge as leaders, and fulfil a leadership role which may be aimed at enabling the group to perform a particular group task (e.g. a department superintendent) or a leader may concentrate more on retaining the cohesion of the group (e.g. personnel officer).

Norms of behaviour vary enormously between cultures, so that an aspect of behaviour which is accepted in one culture may cause extreme offence in another culture.

Communication between adults is largely verbal in most cultures, but eye contact, facial expression and bodily gestures are now recognized as playing an extremely important part in 'body language'. Subtle cues from patients may reveal important information to a keen observer. Such cues existed before the development of language.

Stress, tension and anxiety are usually associated with physiological changes in the activity of the autonomic nervous system, adrenal gland secretion, and other chemical changes, such as the balance of intra-cellular and extra cellular sodium. This affects the excitability of nerve fibres. Ability to respond to stress in this manner is a necessary body defence mechanism, but if such changes are prolonged they can contribute to disorders of the heart, digestive system, and other organic structures. Stress is frequently a contributory factor in rheumatoid arthritis.

A patient's reaction to sickness or injury may take the form of depression, regression of behaviour to a more childish disposition, or, if compensation is involved, a determination to avoid full recovery. It is a mistake to assume that such changes are always intentional. They are better regarded as symptoms which can be corrected by operant conditioning and instilling motivation to improvement.

Details of Psychiatric disorders are outside the scope of this chapter.

International Classification of mental disorders groups them under three headings:

1. Psychoses including schizophrenia, manic-depressive reactions, involutional melancholia, paranoia and paranoid states, senile and pre-senile psychoses, psychosis with cerebral arterio-sclerosis and alcoholic psychosis.

2. Psychoneurotic Disorders including anxiety reaction, hysterical reaction, phobic reaction, neurotic depressive reaction, obsessive-compulsive reaction and various forms of psycho-neuroses with somatic symptoms.

3. Disorders of character, behaviour and intelligence, including pathological personality, immature personality, alcoholism, other drug addictions, primary childhood behaviour disorders and mental deficiency.

As the science of neuropsychology advances more behaviour disorders are recognized as having an organic basis in faulty metabolism or nerve function.

FURTHER READING

Argyle, M. (1967) *The Psychology of Interpersonal Behaviour*.
  Harmondsworth: Penguin.
Beard, R. M. (1969) *An Outline of Piaget's Developmental Psychology*.
  London: Routledge & Kegan Paul.
Eysenck, H. J. (1970) *Fact and Fiction in Psychology*. Harmondsworth:
  Penguin.
Eysenck, H. J. (1953) *Uses and Abuses of Psychology*.
  Harmondsworth: Penguin.
Eysenck, H. J. (1964) *Sense and Nonsense in Psychology*.
  Harmondsworth: Penguin.
Gillis, L. (1972) *Human Behaviour in Illness*. London: Faber & Faber.
Hilgard, E. R., Atkinson, R. C. & Atkinson, R. Z. (1975)
  Introduction to Psychology. London: Harcourt.
Hill, D. A. (1974) *Psychology Teaching*. **2**, 2. Association for the
  Teaching of Psychology.
Hill, D. A. (1977) *Neurology for Physiotherapists*. 2nd edition, ed.
  J. Cash Ch. 22. London: Faber & Faber.
Holding, D. H. (1965) *Principles of Training*. Oxford: Pergamon.
Shakespeare, R. (1975) *The Psychology of Handicap*. London:
  Methuen.
Sheridan, M. D. (1975) *Children's Developmental Progress*. London:
  NFER Publishing Co.
Singh, M. M. (1967) *Mental Disorder*. London: Pan.
Wright, D. S. & Taylor, A. (1972) *Introducing Psychology*.
  Harmondsworth: Penguin.

General pathology

CAUSE OF DISEASE
Congenital
1. Genetic
2. Developmental

Infections
1. Bacteria
2. Virus
3. Fungi
4. Parasites

Infection spread by air, ingestion, direct invasion through skin

Ischaemia

Trauma
1. Fractures
2. Wounds
3. Contusions

Physical agents
1. Temperature
2. Radiation
3. Electric Shock
4. Increased/decreased atmospheric pressure

Chemical
1. Accidental/purposeful ingestion
2. Industrial hazards

Stress
1. Physical
2. Mental

Deficiency
1. Mineral
2. Vitamin

Drugs

DEFENCE MECHANISMS OF THE BODY

1. Skin
2. Mucous membranes
3. Antibodies/immunoglobins
4. Leucocytes

INFLAMMATION

Cause see page 36.

CHANGES IN ACUTE INFLAMMATION

Vascular changes
1. Initial vasoconstriction
2. Succeeded by vasodilitation
3. Stasis
4. Axial stream broadens
5. Margination of leucocytes

Formation of inflammatory exudate
1. Loss of plasma and plasma proteins into tissues
2. Diapedesis of WBC into tissues
3. Chemotaxis to site of injury

WBC – phagocytose bacteria and debris; produce antitoxins
1. Neutrophils – First line defence, phagocytosis
2. Eosinophils – Increase in allergic reactions
3. Basophils – Contain heparin cf. mast cells
4. Monocytes/Histiocytes: Second line defence, remove tissue debris
5. Lymphocytes – Later stage inflammation

ISOLATION OF INFLAMMATORY ACTION

Fibrin formation
1. Limits spread of infection
2. Forms 'scaffolding' for repair
3. Forms adhesions

Spread of infection
1. Lymphatics
2. Blood circulation

SIGNS AND SYMPTOMS OF ACUTE INFLAMMATION

Classical signs
1. Redness
2. Heat
3. Swelling
4. Pain
5. Loss of function

Pathological process
1. Vasodilitation
2. Vasodilitation
3. Inflammatory exudate
4. Tissue damage
5. Oedema/tissue loss

TERMINATION OF ACUTE INFLAMMATION

Resolution — complete restoration of tissue
Involves removal of
1. Inflammatory exudate
2. Fibrin
3. Tissue debris

Suppuration
Due to presence of pyogenic organisms
Leads to formation pus

Abcess
Cavity produced by tissue destruction
If filled with pus drains to nearest surface, or tracks on fascial planes

Chronic inflammation — low grade inflammatory response to minor injury

Divisions
1. Chronic inflammation supervening on acute
2. Chronic inflammation *ab initio*

HEALING AND REPAIR

Occurs after
1. Causative micro-organisms controlled
2. Inflammatory exudate removed

Events
1. Granulation tissue
2. Scar tissue replaces specialized tissues
3. Repair of bone, skin and blood vessels

HAEMORRHAGE

Causes
1. Tissue injuries
2. Pregnancy
3. Childbirth
4. Ulcers
5. Varicose veins
6. Aneurysms

Effects
1. Loss of blood
2. Rise in heart rate
3. Fall in BP

Haemostasis and Clotting
1. Vasoconstriction
2. Thromboplastin formation
3. Conversion prothrombin to thrombin
4. Conversion of fibrinogen to fibrin

SHOCK

Signs and symptoms
1. Pallor
2. Coldness
3. Sweating
4. Nausea/Vomiting
5. Loss consciousness

Caused by reduced cardiac output due to
1. Acute heart failure
2. Oligaemia
3. Pulmonary embolism
4. Infection
5. Anaphylaxis
6. Vasovagal attack

Principles of treatment
1. Lie flat
2. Maintain airway and cardiac output
3. Nothing by mouth if unconscious
4. Call for medical help

OEDEMA

An accumulation of excess fluid in tissue spaces

Mechanism of oedema formation
1. Venous congestion
2. Lymphatic obstruction
3. Hypoproteinaemia
4. Increased capillary permeability
5. Sodium retention
6. Trauma
7. Paralysis
8. Muscle disuse

Principles of treatment
1. Remove cause if possible
2. Increase absorption of fluid by lymphatics
3. Mobilize joints
4. Strengthen muscle
5. Regain normal function

THROMBUS FORMATION – SIMILAR TO BLOOD CLOT, GRADUALLY OCCLUDES VESSEL

1. Common sites
   (i) Coronary aa
   (ii) Cerebral aa
   (iii) Aorta
   (iv) Iliac aa
   (v) Leg veins
2. Cause
   (i) Atheroma
   (ii) Sepsis
3. Sequence of thrombus
   (i) Embolus
   (ii) Resolution and recanalization

EMBOLUS – SOURCE OFTEN OBSCURE

Types
1. Thrombus
2. Fat
3. Air
4. Amniotic fluid

Effect is to block blood vessel(s) causing stasis

DEGENERATION AND NECROSIS

Type	Cause	Tissues affected
1. Cloudy	Toxins, anoxia Inorganic poisons	Heart, liver, kidney
2. Fatty	Toxins, ischaemia Chlorinated hydrocarbons	Heart, liver, kidney
3. Necrosis	Toxins, infarction	All tissues
4. Gangrene	Toxins, ischaemia	Limbs, lung, intestines

HYPERTROPHY AND HYPERPLASIA

Hypertrophy
1. Increase in cell size
2. Occurs in tissues which cannot reproduce

Hyperplasia
1. Increase in cell numbers
2. Occurs in cells which reproduce

Cause of both
1. Hormones
2. 'Extra work'

ATROPHY

1. Antithesis of hypertrophy and hyperplasia
2. Caused by starvation, ischaemia and disuse

NEOPLASM

Cancer is disordered cell growth

Cause
1. Genetic
2. Environmental
3. Hormonal
4. Virus
5. Chemical carcinogens
6. Radiation

Spread by
1. Lymphatics
2. Blood
3. Invasive growth

Microscopic appearance
1. Epidermoid carcinoma (skin tissues)
2. Adenocarcinoma (lymphoid tissue)
3. Anaplastic — without parent tissue likeness
4. Differentiated — some parents tissue likeness

Sites
1. Skin
2. Mouth
3. Lung
4. Stomach
5. Breast
6. Uterus

FURTHER READING

Boyd, W. (1971) *Introduction to the Study of Disease*. Philadelphia: Lea & Febiger.

Hurley, J. V. (1972) *Acute Inflammation*. Edinburgh: Churchill Livingstone.

Ward, F. A. (1977) *Primer of Pathology*. London: Butterworth.

Diseases of joints

CLASSIFICATION

GROUP A   Arthritis of unknown cause
GROUP B   Arthritis due to infection
GROUP C   Degenerative joint disease
GROUP D   Crystal arthritis
GROUP E   Connective tissue diseases

GROUP A   ARTHRITIS OF UNKNOWN CAUSE

RHEUMATOID ARTHRITIS

Systemic disease. Ranges from few joints mildly affected to complete ankylosis, and bed-ridden state. Age of onset puberty to old age. Two thirds before age 50.

Signs and symptoms
1. Polyarthritis, often symmetrical
2. Small joints in hands and feet affected first (particularly metacarpo-phalangeal and proximal interphalangeal joints)
3. Pain on movement
4. Morning stiffness of variable duration
5. Synovial thickening
6. Joints inflamed, painful and tender
7. Loss of range of movement
8. Flexion contractures
9. Finger deformities;
    (i)   Swan neck
    (ii) Ulnar deviation
    (iii) Boutonnière
    (iv) Subluxation
10. Clawed toes and callosities under MT heads
11. Valgus ankles
12. Generally valgus knees
13. Rheumatoid nodules on extensor surfaces
14. Thin skin
15. General malaise

Radiographic features
1. Soft tissue swellings
2. Osteoporosis
3. Loss of joint space
4. Bone erosions
5. Subluxation and deformity
6. Bony ankylosis

Pathological changes
1. Joints
   - (i)   Synovial inflammation and proliferation
   - (ii)   Cartilage and bone erosions
   - (iii) Cyst formation in bone
   - (iv)   Bone loss
   - (v)   Inflammation of synovial tendon sheaths
   - (vi)   Erosion and rupture of tendons
   - (vii) Large synovial cysts − e.g. behind knee
2. Vascular changes:
   - (i)   Small arteries occluded
   - (ii)   Ulcers
   - (iii) Neuropathies sensory and motor
3. Nerve entrapment:
   - (i)   At carpal tunnel
   - (ii)   Behind elbow
   - (iii) Round fibula head
4. Chest:
   - (i)   Nodules in lung
   - (ii)   Pleural effusions
   - (iii) Interstitial fibrosis
5. Eye:
   - (i)   Inflammatory changes
   - (ii)   Dry eyes (Sjogren's syndrome)
   - (iii) Sight impairment
6. General:
   - (i)   Nodule formation
   - (ii)   Anaemia
   - (iii) Elevated erythrocyte sedimentation rate
   - (iv)   Positive rheumatoid factor tests in 70 per cent cases
   - (v)   Atlanto-axial subluxation
   - (vi)   Amyloidosis
   - (vii) Renal involvement
   - (viii) Skin thinning
   - (ix)   Weight loss
   - (x)   Osteoporosis

Assessment

Observe
1. General appearance
2. Gait
3. Apparent age
4. Cleanliness of body and clothes

Enquire
1. Actual age
2. Duration and severity of illness
3. Sites of pain
4. Special difficulties
5. Home circumstances
6. Work circumstances
7. Family commitments
8. People/Services already assisting
9. Drug therapy

Examination
1. All joints for heat, tenderness and swelling
2. Range of all movements
3. Assess motor power
4. Feet for callosities

Assess
1. Likely response to treatment
2. Help required from other agencies

Principles of management

General
1. Drug therapy must be adequate
2. Working against pain does not increase muscle power
3. Over-exertion should be avoided

Acute stage — pain relief
1. Anti-inflammatory and analgesic drugs
2. Rest acutely painful joints
3. Use splints if necessary
4. Bed rest for polyarthritis
5. Ice packs

Sub-acute — increase mobility
1. Ice packs
2. Gentle active movements
3. Isometric contractions
4. Hydrotherapy
5. Weight bearing after muscle control is achieved
6. Avoid sticks, crutches etc., to preserve upper limb joints

Chronic stage
1. Encourage mobility
2. Increase muscle power
3. Give necessary walking aids
4. Advise on self care

Treatment methods

Pain relief
1. Rest
2. Ice packs or 2 lb bags of frozen peas. Latter are reuseable
3. Wax, e.g. for hands
4. Heat, but not for inflamed joints
5. Resting splints. Plaster of Paris or plastazote

Mobilizing
1. Exercises within pain-free range
2. Particular attention to neck and shoulder girdle
3. Suspension exercises
4. Spring assisted or lightly resisted exercise
5. Pendular exercises
6. Hydrotherapy

Strengthening
1. Graduated isometric exercise
2. Introduce isotonic exercise
3. Pay particular attention to postural muscles

Advice
1. Adequate rest
2. Housework programme
3. Home exercise programme
4. Keep weight down
5. If necessary
   (i) Alter furniture
   (ii) Provide handrails
   (iii) Provide walking aids and splints
   (iv) Change employment

After initial treatment re-assess
1. Residual disability
2. Patient's disposition
3. Attitude to disease
4. Relationship with family and workmates
5. Ability and desire to respond to treatment
6. Advisability of further therapy

Surgical treatment
In suitable cases a programme may include:
1. Synovectomy
2. Excision arthroplasty
3. Interposition arthroplasty
4. Partial or total joint replacement
5. Arthrodesis

Where operative treatment not indicated
Appropriate aids may include:
1. Supportive splints
   (i)   Wrists: Orthoplast or polythene
   (ii) Knees: Glassona, polythene or metal caliper
   (iii) Ankles: Polythene or metal caliper
2. Walking aids: Sticks, crutches, light pick-ups
3. Special shoes of soft leather incorporating
   (i)   Insoles
   (ii) Heel flares
   (iii) Raises or wedges
4. Wheelchairs

JUVENILE RHEUMATOID ARTHRITIS

Several types:
One or two large joints affected
Polyarthritis similar to adults
Polyarthritis with systemic illness
Polyarthritis leading to ankylosing spondylitis
Peak age of onset 2–4 years
Second peak before puberty
Only 5 per cent carry disease to adulthood

Signs and symptoms
1. Joint inflammation
2. Onset larger joints
3. Spinal involvement
4. Tendency to ankylosis
5. Eye inflammation
6. Rheumatoid factor test usually negative

Principles of management
1. Relieve pain
2. Prevent deformity
3. Maintain mobility
4. Prolonged immobilization inadvisable
5. Education must be kept up

Treatment methods:
1. Adequate analgesia (especially preceding physical treatment)
2. Ice packs
3. Hydrotherapy of especial value
4. Active exercises for mobility
5. Correct positioning in bed
6. Postural exercises
7. Short term splintage of inflamed joints

ANKYLOSING SPONDYLITIS

Sexes affected equally
Males more severely
Onset 16–40 years

Signs and symptoms
1. Lumbar backache
2. Pain and stiffness after rest
3. Sacro-iliac joints tender to forced movement
4. Stiff back
5. Loss of lumbar curve
6. Progressive thoracic kyphosis
7. Forward extended head
8. Reduced chest expansion
9. Sunken chest and pot belly
10. Hips and shoulders may become involved
11. Plantar fasciitis
12. Achilles tendonitis

Radiographic features
1. Sacro-iliac erosion and later fusion
2. Arthritic changes in apophyseal joints
3. Ligamentous ossification in spine
4. Squaring of vertebral bodies
5. New bone growth between vertebrae ('syndesmophytes')
6. Peripheral joint erosions

Pathological changes
1. Ligamentous and capsular inflammation
2. Synovial inflammation
3. Ossification
4. Ankylosis
5. Rheumatoid factor tests negative
6. ESR raised

Complications
1. Reduced chest expansion and vital capacity
2. Possibility of chest infection
3. Atlanto-axial subluxation
4. Possible cord damage
5. Fractures of rigid spine
6. 10 per cent cases have iritis
7. Associated ulcerative bowel disease

Assessment

Measure:
1. Finger-floor distance, standing with straight knees
2. Chest expansion below nipple line
3. Occiput-wall distance, standing with heels to wall
4. Schroeber's index, i.e. mark 4/5 lumbar space, mark 10 cm upwards, Measure between marks on forward flexion
5. Vital capacity
6. Range of other joint movement

Principles of management
1. Maintain and increase spinal mobility
2. Prevent and correct deformity
3. Increase chest expansion and vital capacity
4. Attention to posture
5. Drug therapy for relief of pain and stiffness
6. Advice to patient

Treatment methods

Pain relief
Analgesics and anti-inflammatory drugs

Mobilizing
1. Vigorous exercises including
   (i) Side flexion
   (ii) Rotation
   (iii) Extension of all parts of the spine
2. Breathing exercises
3. Chest mobility exercises
4. Hip and shoulder exercises
5. Shoulder girdle exercises

Strengthening
1. Back extension exercises
2. Postural exercises
Give short course of supervised treatment
Teach home exercises
Re-assess in one month
Treat if necessary
Thereafter re-assess yearly

Advice to patients
1. Instruct concerning the nature of the disease
2. Emphasize importance of daily exercise
3. Put a board under mattress
4. Use one pillow or none
5. Spend some time prone lying daily
6. Supine lying if prone impossible
7. Perform home exercises twice daily
8. Always be conscious of posture

Adjust if necessary
Height of work bench or desk
Chair
Teach best method of performing daily tasks

REITERS DISEASE

A combination of urethritis and arthritis
Attacks young men
Usually develops from sexually transmitted non-specific urethritis
May follow dysentry
The venereal type rare in women

Signs and symptoms
1. Urethral discharge: dysuria
2. Acute arthritis follows in 10–21 days
3. Arthritis commonly affects knees, ankles and feet
4. Other peripheral joints may be affected
5. Systemic reaction
6. Fever
7. Weight loss
8. General malaise
9. Conjunctivitis with sterile eye discharge (40 per cent)
10. Mouth and genital ulceration (10 per cent)
11. Keratoderma blennorrhagica on hands and feet (10 per cent)

Radiographic features
Similar to rheumatoid arthritis

Pathological changes
1. Urethritis
2. Synovial proliferation and effusion
3. Tendonitis around ankle
4. Plantar fascitis
5. Erosive arthritis
6. Genital and mouth ulceration
7. Reiter's cells (large macrophages) in synovial fliud

Principles of management
1. Treat venereal disease
2. Acute arthritic symptoms treated as for rheumatoid arthritis
3. Surgery may become necessary in persistent or recurrent cases
4. Advice about re-infection and disease recurrence

Treatment methods
1. Oxy-tetracyline for urethritis
2. Anti-inflammatory drugs
3. Joint aspiration
4. Intra-articular injection of steroids
5. Bed rest with splints if necessary
6. Ice packs
7. Graduated active exercises, especially quadriceps
8. Weight bearing when good muscle control is established

PSORIATIC ARTHROPATHY

Psoriasis. May be small skin or scalp patches
Nail pitting and ridging
Little systemic upset
Rheumatoid factor tests negative
Varied joint disease
(i)   Erosive terminal joint disease in hands and feet
(ii) Polyarthritis but less symmetrical than rheumatoid arthritis. Flexor tendon involvement
(iii) Sacro-iliac and spinal arthritis
(iv) Rare, destructive arthritis mutilans in hands and feet
Treatment as for rheumatoid arthritis

GROUP B   ARTHRITIS DUE TO INFECTION

RHEUMATIC FEVER

A disease of decreasing incidence and severity
Affects young people

Signs and symptoms
1. Fever
2. Infection of the throat
3. Skin rash
4. Transient polyarthritis
5. Subcutaneous nodules
6. General malaise

Pathological changes
1. Streptococcal infection
2. Inflammatory synovitis of joints
3. Inflammatory damage to the heart
4. Cardiac arrhythmias
5. Mitral or aortic valve disease
6. Possible permanent heart damage
7. Produces disability at times of cardiac strain, e.g. pregnancy

Principles of management
1. Drug therapy
2. Bed rest
3. No need for splints
4. Progressive mobilization

Treatment methods

Acute stage:
1. Antibiotics for streptococcal infection
2. Analgesic and anti-inflammatory drugs
3. Bed rest
4. Ice packs
5. Gentle active movements

Subacute stage:
1. Progressive mobilization
2. Graduated active exercise
3. Paliative ice or heat
4. Suspension exercises
5. Hydrotherapy

Chronic stage
1. Prophylactic long-term antibiotics
2. Assessment of cardiac damage
3. Advice about activity levels

SEPTIC ARTHRITIS

Bacterial infection of joint introduced by operation, trauma or injection
May spread from infection elsewhere
Metal prostheses may attract bacteria

Signs and symptoms
1. Any joint may be affected, usually monoarticular
2. Acutely painful
3. Inflamed
4. Fever
5. Raised erythrocyte sedimentation rate
6. Commonly, staphylococcal infection

Principles of management
1. Identify source of infection
2. Bacteriological culture of synovial fluid and blood
3. Suitable antibiotics
4. Surgical drainage if necessary
5. Rest, often with splints
6. Later mobilization
Arthritis may also occur in association with other infections
1. Gonorrhoea
2. Brucellosis
3. Tuberculosis
4. Erythema nodosum
5. Some virus diseases
6. Ulcerative colitis

GROUP C   DEGENERATIVE JOINT DISEASE

MONOARTICULAR OSTEOARTHROSIS

A disease of large synovial joints
Attacks both sexes equally
Middle age onwards
Possible genetic influence

Signs and symptoms
1.   Hip and knee joints most commonly attacked
2.   Pain on movement
3.   Later rest pain
4.   Night pain
5.   Sometimes referred pain
6.   Muscle spasm
7.   Progressive loss of range of movement
8.   Joint stiffness after rest
9.   Moderate effusion
10. Thickened joints
11. Crepitus; sometimes audible
12. Hip deformity, usually
     (i)   Adduction
     (ii) Flexion
     (iii) Outward rotation
13. Knee deformity usually
     (i)   Varus
     (ii) Flexion
14. Leg length discrepancy due to fixed flexion

Radiographic features
1.   Diminished joint space
2.   Sclerosis of subchondral bone
3.   Cysts in subchondral bone
4.   New bone growth: osteophytes
5.   Loose bodies
6.   Subluxation of joint

Pathological changes
1. Softening and fibrillation of articular cartilage
2. Thinning of articular cartilage
3. Complete loss of cartilage
4. Subchondral bone sclerosis
5. Contracture of capsule
6. Mild synovial reaction
7. Calcification of ligamentous attachments
8. Calcification of cartilage and loose bodies
9. Cyst formation in bone
10. Bone infarction
11. Collapse of joint surfaces
12. Subluxation of joint
13. Bony ankylosis

Precipitating pathology may be
1. Obesity
2. Congenital abnormalities
3. Perthé's disease and related bone damage in adolescents
4. Rheumatoid or other arthritis
5. Trauma
6. Fracture

Assessment
Keep careful records

Observe:
1. General appearance
2. Gait
3. If stick or walking aid used
4. If overweight

Enquire
1. Site and duration of pain
2. If night pain
3. If precipitated by other pathology
4. Special difficulties
5. Nature of employment

Examination
Hip joint
1. Measure range of movement
   (i)   Active
   (ii) Passive
2. Measure leg lengths for
   (i)   True
   (ii) Apparent shortening
3. Palpate for
   (i)   Tender areas
   (ii) Muscle spasm
4. Assess power of all muscle groups
5. Carry out Trendelenberg test

Other joints
1. Observe redness and swelling
2. Palpate for
   (i)   Heat
   (ii) Tenderness
   (iii) Muscle spasm
3. Measure joint circumference
4. Measure range of movement
   (i)   Active
   (ii) Passive
5. Assess muscle power
6. Compare with contralateral joint

Principles of management
1. Pain relief
2. Increase mobility
3. Increase muscle power
4. Surgical treatment
5. Advice on self-care

Treatment methods

To reduce pain and muscle spasm
1. Drug therapy
2. Ice packs
3. Shortwave diathermy
   Caution Heat treatment may aggravate symptoms
4. Ultrasound
5. Hydrotherapy
6. Suspension exercises

To mobilize
1. Passive mobilizations 'Maitlands'
2. Positioning of patient, e.g. prone lying
3. Pulley exercises
4. Traction
5. Suspension exercises
6. Active movements
7. Hydrotherapy

To increase muscle power
1. Proprioceptive neuromuscular facilitation techniques
2. Isometric and isotonic exercises
3. Pulley exercises
4. Weight resisted exercises

To improve function
1. Postural exercises
2. Gait training
3. Supply if required;

    (i) Walking aids
    (ii) Splints made of: Plastazote
                                Plaster of Paris
                                Glassona
                                Polythene
    (iii) Footwear. Incorporating: Insoles
                                Heel flares
                                Heel cups
                                Wedges
    (iv) Calipers

Surgical treatment
1. Osteotomy
2. Excision arthroplasty
3. Interposition arthroplasty
4. Partial or total joint replacement
5. Arthrodesis
For post-operative management see orthopaedic section

Advice to patient
1. Diet and weight control
2. Home exercises
3. Use of walking aids
4. Use of household aids
5. Adaptation of furniture
Re-assess patient and review treatment at intervals

GENERALIZED OSTEOARTHROSIS

Attacks the middle aged to elderly
Women more than men
Strong genetic influence

Signs and symptoms
1. Characteristic bony swellings on terminal phalanges (Heberden nodes)
2. Painful polyarthritis
3. Joints become tender and thickened
4. May be inflamed
5. Joint stiffness
6. Painful joints
7. Progressive loss of range of movement
8. Fine crepitus
9. Deformity

Joints most commonly affected
  (i)   Distal inter-phalangeal of hands
  (ii) First carpometacarpal
  (iii) Other joints of hand
  (iv) Knee
Radiographic and pathological changes as in monoarticular osteoarthrosis

Assessment
As for monoarticular disease

Principles of management
As for monoarticular disease
Surgery is less frequently indicated except for first carpometacarpal joint

CERVICO-LUMBAR SPONDYLOSIS AND DISC DEGENERATION

Affects adults past middle age
Depression is often a feature

Cervical spine

Signs and symptoms

Apophyseal joints
1. Neck pain. Aggravated by movement
2. Stiffness
3. Limitation of movement
4. Crepitus

Intervertebral discs
Commonly C5–7 level
1. Aching pain
2. Increasing to severe pain
3. Limitation of movement

Nerve root compression
1. Radiating pain
2. Paraesthesia
3. Decreased reflexes in root distribution
4. Muscle weakness

Cord compression
Increased leg reflexes

Vertebral artery compression
Movement precipitates
1. Visual disturbances
2. Transient blackouts

LUMBAR SPINE

Signs and symptoms

Apophyseal joints
Less frequently affected:
1. Pain aggravated by movement
2. Rigid back
3. Limited movements

Intervertebral discs
Usually L 4–5 or L 5–S1 level
1. Low back pain
2. Aggravated by coughing or sneezing
3. Sciatic pain increased by nerve stretching
4. Muscle spasm
5. Scoliosis
6. Loss of lumbar curve
7. Flexion limited

Nerve root compression
1. Radiating pain
2. Paraesthesia
3. Numbness
4. Diminished or absent reflexes
5. Muscle weakness

Cauda Equina compression
1. Back pain
2. Bilateral radiating pain
3. Bilateral paralysis
4. Bilateral sensory loss
5. Loss of sphincter control

ACUTE DISC LESIONS

Usually traumatic in origin
Affect a younger more active age group

Signs and symptoms
1. Sudden acute onset
2. Severe pain
3. Spasm
4. Scoliosis
5. Loss of spinal movement

Nerve root and cord compression symptoms
As described above but more acute

Radiographic features
X-ray changes do not necessarily correlate with symptoms, especially in cervical region
1. Reduced joint spaces
2. Reduced disc spaces
3. Arthritic changes in apophyseal joints
4. Bone sclerosis
5. Alteration of normal spinal curves
6. Scoliosis
7. Osteophyte formation
8. Myelogram may show disc protrusion and nerve root compression

Pathological changes

Degenerative disease
1. Osteoarthrotic changes in joints
2. Degenerative changes in annulus fibrosus
3. Extrusion of nuclear pulposus
4. Bone cyst formation
5. Osteophyte formation
6. Kinking of vertebral arteries

Traumatic disease
1. Tear of vertebral muscles
2. Tear of interspinal ligaments
3. Apophyseal joint subluxation
4. Disc prolapse

Assessment
1. Medical and radiographic investigations must first be carried out
2. Obtain accurate history
3. Examination:
   - (i) Presence of spasm and scoliosis
   - (ii) Palpate for tenderness
   - (iii) Range of movement in all planes
   - (iv) Effect of movement
     - a. Active
     - b. Passive
   - (v) Appropriate nerve stretch tests
   - (vi) Test sensation

Principles of management

Pain relief
1. Analgesics
2. Rest
3. Heat
4. Traction
5. Passive manipulation

Spinal support
1. Plaster jacket or corset
2. Cervical collar

Postural re-education

Advise patient on self-care

Surgical intervention
To decompress nerve roots or cord
(i) Laminectomy
(ii) Discectomy
(iii) Spinal fusion

Treatment methods

Acute stages
1. Analgesics
2. Bed rest. Possibly prolonged
3. Heat packs
4. Head traction for cervical lesions
5. Pelvic or leg traction for lumbar lesions
6. Careful manipulation

Subacute stage
1. Local heat. Infra red. Short wave diathermy
2. Passive mobilizations
3. Careful active movements
4. Exercises:
   Neck
   Shoulder girdle
   Abdomen
   Leg extension
5. Support if required
   (i) Cervical collar appropriately firm
   (ii) Corset or plaster jacket
6. Careful manipulation

Recovery stage
1. Work towards full mobility
2. Progressively vigorous exercises for
   (i) Spine; all sections
   (ii) Shoulder girdle
   (iii) Abdominal wall
   (iv) Pelvic girdle
   (v) Legs
3. Advice
   (i) Simple regime of home exercises
   (ii) Board under mattress
   (iii) Lifting techniques
   (iv) Avoidance of strain
   (v) Suitable sport and activity
   (vi) Suitable chair at home and work
   (vii) Adaptation of work situation

GROUP D   CRYSTAL ARTHRITIS

GOUT

Affects adult males
Women after menopause

Signs and symptoms
1. Severe pain cf. septic arthritis
2. Local inflammation
3. Any joint. Usually monarticular
4. Commonest in 1st MTP joint
5. Uncommon in hip or shoulder

Pathological changes
1. In joint
   (i) Inflammatory
   (ii) Often violent reaction
   (iii) Uric acid crystals in synovial fluid
2. Systemic
   (i) Raised plasma uric acid
   (ii) Raised white cell count
3. Complications
   (i) Tophi, urate deposits in soft tissues
   (ii) Secondary degenerative arthritis
   (iii) Renal disease

Medical treatment

Drug therapy
   (i) Indomethacin, Phenylbutazone for acute attack
   (ii) Allopurinol for long term prevention
Physiotherapy not usually indicated

PSEUDO-GOUT

Affects either sex
Usually over 45 years

Signs and symptoms
1. Usually monoarticular
2. Commonly knee, shoulder or wrist
3. Joint hot, tender, swollen and painful
4. Synovial effusion
5. Occasionally insidious and polyarticular cf. Rheumatoid arthritis
6. Occasionally insidious and cause of osteoarthrosis

Medical treatment
1. Analgesic and anti-inflammatory drugs
2. Joint aspiration
3. Intra-articular corticosteroid injections

Physiotherapy treatment
1. Ice packs
2. Early mobilization
3. Restoration of muscle strength and bulk
4. Weight bearing exercises

GROUP E   CONNECTIVE TISSUE DISEASES

SCLERODERMA

A rare progressive disease of unknown cause

Signs and symptoms
1. Raynaud's phenomenon
2. Tight shiny skin
3. Sclerodactyly
4. Telangectasia
5. Calcinosis
6. Slightly swollen joints
7. Loss of range of movement
8. Skin ulceration
9. Oesophageal stricture

Pathological changes
1. Increased collagen production
2. Skin tethering
3. Fibrosis of lungs, kidneys and other organs
4. Mild synovitis

Complications
1. Hypertension
2. Malnutrition
3. Heart and lung failure

Principles of management
1. Treat complications
2. Encourage mobility
3. Drugs of doubtful value

Treatment methods
1. Drug therapy
2. Wax for hands and feet
3. Gentle passive stretching
4. Active movements
5. Ulcer care including ultraviolet light

Advice to patient
1. Keep extremities warm
2. Regular daily exercise

OTHER CONNECTIVE TISSUE DISEASES ARE:

1. Dermatomyositis
2. Disseminated lupus erythematosis
3. Polymyalgia rheumatica
4. Polyarteritis nodosa

FURTHER READING

Boyle, J. Buchanan, W. W. (1971) *Clinical Rheumatology*. London: Blackwell.
Cash, J. E. ed. (1976) *A textbook of Medical Conditions for Physiotherapists*. London: Faber & Faber.
Day, B. H. (1972) *Orthopaedic Appliances*. London: Faber & Faber.
Goble, R. E. A. & Nicholls, P. J. R. (1971) *Rehabilitation of Severely Disabled*. Vols 1 and 2, London: Butterworth.
Hollander, J. L. & McCarthy, D. J. eds. (1972) *Arthritis and Allied Conditions A Textbook of Rheumatology*. Philadelphia: Lea & Febiger.
Mason, M. & Currey, H. L. F. eds. (1970) *An Introduction to Clinical Rheumatology*. London: Pitman.
Scott, J. T. ed. (1977) *Textbook of Rheumatic Diseases*. Edinburgh: Churchill Livingstone.

General surgery: respiratory and cardiac diseases

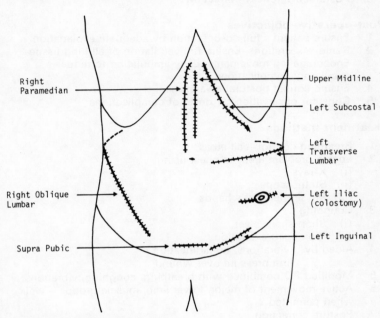

Right Paramedian

Upper Midline

Left Subcostal

Left Transverse Lumbar

Right Oblique Lumbar

Left Iliac (colostomy)

Supra Pubic

Left Inguinal

Fig. 1. Common abdominal incisions

COMMON COMPLICATIONS OF GENERAL SURGERY

1. Respiratory complications e.g. atelectasis
2. Circulatory complications e.g. phlebothrombosis
3. Haemorrhage
4. Muscle imbalance/atrophy – worse in the elderly and debilitated patient
5. Unhealed wounds
6. Incisional hernia (see Fig. 1)

PHYSIOTHERAPY

Pre-operative principles
Assess respiratory competence to determine need for
1. Breathing exercises – stress areas most affected by the surgery
2. Effective coughing
3. Postural drainage (PD) – modified to particular patient
4. Foot/leg movements – aimed to aid circulation
5. Postural awareness/correction

Post-operative objectives
1. Ensure patient's full co-operation by adequate explanation
2. Remove secretions. Ensure full ventilation of all lung tissue
3. Encourage leg movements. Early ambulation to reduce circulatory complications
4. Ensure correct postural awareness
5. Constant observation for onset of complications

Treatment methods
1. Breathing control – all areas
2. Locate problem areas in chest using
   (i) X-rays
   (ii) Stethoscope
   (iii) Physiotherapist's hands
3. Coughing
   (i) Short sharp blast
   (ii) Prolonged expiration
4. Aided by – vibrations, humidification or firm pressure over wound
5. Modified PD combined with breathing, coughing, vibrations
6. Active movement of major, lower limb, muscle groups – walk when permitted
7. Posture correction
8. Abdominal muscle contractions – static/active

CHEST AND HEART DISEASE

Important factors for consideration

Cyanosis
1. Peripheral
2. Central

Apex beat — position

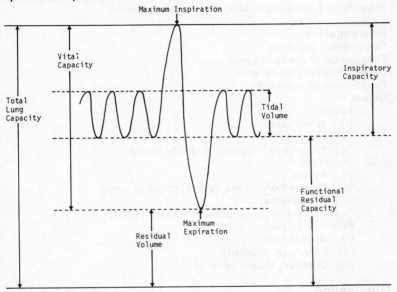

Fig. 2. Lung volumes

Minute ventilation — tidal volume × respiratory rate per minute

Lung compliance — a measure of lung elasticity

Diffusion defects — here arterial pO_2, pCO_2 values are relatively normal at rest but decreased with exercise, as in emphysema, etc.

Blood gas analysis — in the normal resting adult, arterial blood gas values are
1. $pCO_2 = 35 - 45$ mmHg (4.7 – 6.0 kPa)
2. $pO_2 = 80 - 100$ mmHg (11.3 – 14.00 kPa)
   (kPa = kilopascal, kPa × 7.5 = mmHg)

Oxygen therapy — in chronic hypoxia from hypoventilation (e.g. chronic bronchitis) only low concentration oxygen therapy should be given, unless ventilation is assisted ('anoxic state' drives the respiratory centre). In hypoxia from impaired gaseous exchange (e.g. pneumonia) high concentration oxygen therapy can be safely administered

MEDICAL CHEST CONDITIONS:
PHYSIOTHERAPY ASSESSMENT FOR PATIENT WITH
CHEST DISEASE

Observation on entry to Department/Ward
Patient must then be adequately supported and undressed

Read notes
Extract relevant information e.g. past medical history, occupation, environment, smoking habits, any heart condition

Interrogation
Symptoms – duration
Time/mode of onset of symptoms
General health/activity levels
Progression of condition
Details of
1. Cough
    (i)   When present
    (ii) Unproductive
    (iii) Productive – quality, quantity, odour
2. Dyspnoea
    (i)   At rest
    (ii) On exertion – note degree/speed of onset
    (iii) Orthopnoea
    (iv) Paroxsysmal nocturnal dyspnoea (PND)
3. Presence of pain
    (i)   Note details
    (ii) Area, type, intensity
    (iii) Duration, means of relief

Observation
1. General health/appearance
    (i)   Weight loss
    (ii) Emaciation
2. Skin colour
    (i)   Cyanosis
    (ii) Pallor
3. Shape of thorax
    (i)   Barrel
    (ii) Kyphosis
    (iii) Flattened areas
4. Abnormal respiratory movements
    (i)   Unilateral breathing
    (ii) Paradoxical movement
    (iii) Shallow breathing
    (iv) Flail segment
    (v)   Accessory muscles
5. Digital clubbing
6. Mediastinal shift denoted by tracheal position

Palpation
1. Tracheal position
2. Chest wall — noting:
   (i) Degree/equality of expansion
   (ii) Areas of diminished movement
   (iii) Tenderness
   (iv) Areas of 'blow out'
3. Supra clavicular lymph nodes
   (i) If enlarged infection/malignancy
4. Apex beat position — displacement may indicate:
   (i) Enlarged heart
   (ii) Pleural effusion
   (iii) Mediastinal shift

Percussion
(i) Dull over collapse/consolidation
(ii) 'Stoney dull' over pleural effusion
(iii) Hyperresonant over pneumothorax

Auscultation
1. Audible — wheeze, stridor, bubbling
2. Stethoscopic — vesicular, bronchial, Râles, rhonchi, pleural rub

Measurements
1. Vitalograph
2. Peak flow
3. Chest expansion — in all areas
4. Range of movement
   (i) Thoracic spine
   (ii) Shoulder joint/girdle
5. Respiratory rate
   (i) At rest
   (ii) On exertion (if practical)
6. Patient's weight

Reading X-rays
1. Compare present/past films
2. Observation for abnormalities/worsening
3. Read reports

CHRONIC BRONCHITIS

Definition
A condition with chronic or recurrent increase, above normal, in the volume of mucus secretion, sufficient to cause expectoration, when other localized broncho pulmonary disease is excluded as the source of the increased expectoration.

When accompanied by widespread bronchospasm, known as chronic obstructive airways disease.

Aetiology
1. Cold damp climate predisposes
2. Common in cigarette smokers
3. Male incidence higher
4. Manifests in middle age onwards – gradual worsening
5. Greater incidence in dusty occupations, urban habitation
6. May be genetically linked

Pathological changes
1. Hypertrophy of mucous glands in trachea/bronchi
2. Goblet cells increase, particularly in bronchioles
3. Increased secretions from mucous glands/goblet cells – thick and sticky
4. Mucous membrane thickened
5. Inhaled irritants→bronchospasm
6. Partial obstruction due to 4 and 5
7. Cilia unable to remove secretions
8. Stagnant secretions→chronic recurrent infection
9. Chronic infection→degeneration – fibrous tissue replaces:
   (i) Epithelial lining
   (ii) Some smooth muscle/cartilaginous tissue
10. Fibrous tissue contracts→compensatory emphysema

Clinical features
1. Insidious onset – years
2. Cough
   (i) Initially – lasts several weeks/minimal respite
                  sputum mucoid, occasionally purulent
   (ii) Later – lasts throughout winter, then all year, sputum
                  quantity increased, periodic acute episodes
   (iii) Advanced – irritating and dry
3. Dyspnoea
4. Cyanosis (hypoventilation)
5. Exercise tolerance decreases
6. Respiratory movements diminished (apical breathing predominates)
7. Arterial pO_2 falls, pCO_2 rises
   (termed as 'blue bloaters' – cyanotic with a barrel chest)

Complications
1. Respiratory failure
2. Corpulmonale
3. Pneumonia
4. Congestive cardiac failure (CCF)

Principles of physiotherapy
Early stages:
1. Prevent respiratory infection — remove secretions
2. Prevent exacerbations by avoiding predisposing situations
3. Improve breathing control — breathing exercises
4. Chemotherapy where appropriate — bronchodilators, antibiotics, linctus
5. Teach effective coughing
6. Improve thoracic mobility/increase exercise tolerance

Treatment methods
Techniques may include modified PD vibration/shaking
Later stages:
as before but emphasis on:
1. Encouragement of relaxation in all positions
2. Elimination of fear
3. Assisting the patient to understand the condition and his role in the treatment regime
4. Encouraging maximum use of lung tissue with minimal effort — often intermittent positive pressure breathing is used (IPPB)
5. Mobilizing secretions, IPPB, vibrations, modified PD
6. Instruction to maintain good postural awareness/control

Acute exacerbation
These patients retain CO_2 and may be drowsy/semi-conscious
1. Establish adequate ventilation/mobilize secretions
2. IPPB using a face mask — coughing/suction as required
3. Administer low concentration oxygen therapy
4. Bronchodilators may be nebulized
With such patients it is unwise to commence continuous artificial ventilation as 'weaning' is difficult

BRONCHIAL ASTHMA

Characterized by variable, often paroxsysmal dyspnoea due to widespread narrowing of bronchioles — intermittent partial airways obstruction
Two types:
1. Extrinsic
2. Intrinsic
In either the attack may be sudden or gradual

Pathological changes

During an attack
1. Bronchospasm
2. Mucosal oedema
3. Viscid secretion forms plugs in medium/small bronchioles

When a mild attack subsides, chest returns to normal as thick mucus is expectorated

Following a severe attack→absorption collapse

Repeated and sustained attacks→hypertrophy mucous membrane and thickening of all layers of smaller bronchi

Both worsen effects of further attacks making expiration more difficult

Signs and symptoms of attack
1. May be warning signs e.g. chest tightens
2. Audible wheezing, expiration difficult
3. Dyspnoea
4. Increased respiratory rate
5. Decreased vital capacity
6. Over use accessory muscles of respiration
7. Distressing unproductive cough

As attack subsides
(i) Bronchospasm ceases
(ii) Productive cough occurs
(iii) Patient is exhausted

Duration of attack variable (5 minutes→24 hours)

Over 24 hours, status asthmaticus is present

Principles of physiotherapy
1. Teach patient to understand, control and manage an attack
2. Reassurance – do not show concern over an attack – firm, sympathetic handling
3. With a child gain parental co-operation and explain their role to maintain a normal active child
4. Instruction on drug self administration e.g. bronchodilators
5. Prevention of long term effects from recurrent attacks
6. Instruction on positions of relaxation – to 'ward off an attack'
7. Encourage prolonged relaxed expiration
8. Aid expectoration
9. Control and maintenance of relaxed breathing during everyday activities
10. Maintain thoracic mobility
11. Improve postural defects

Treatment methods
1. Local/general relaxation – all positions
2. Unilateral/bilateral basal breathing control
3. Relaxed expiration
4. Vibrations/modified PD
5. Expiration/inspiration to counting
6. Strap exercises
7. IPPB – bronchodilators nebulized
8. Assess progress – vitalograph, peak flow, chest measurements

EMPHYSEMA

Condition characterized by enlargement of air spaces distal to the bronchioles, accompanied by destructive changes
Two types:
1. Centrilobular
2. Panlobular
Can occur separately or coexist

Causes
1. Localized
   (i) Congenital
   (ii) Compensatory e.g. secondary to resection
   (iii) Partial bronchial occlusion e.g. neoplasm
2. Generalized
   (i) Secondary to chronic lung disease
   (ii) Occupational/excess lung distension e.g. trumpeter
   (iii) Senile (physiological weakness)

Pathological changes
If from:
1. Partial occlusion/chronic lung disease air flow is obstructed, particularly expiration. Air trapping on expiration, followed by hyper-inflation with inspiration. Walls of terminal airways weaken→breakdown→Bullae formation
2. Regular overdistension – atrophy of small airways→breakdown →Bullae formation
3. Physiological ageing – atrophy of elastic tissue/fibrosis in smaller airways. Distension on inspiration, expiration using accessory muscles→air trapping→septal breakdown→Bullae

Signs and symptoms
1. Progressive dyspnoea/orthopnoea
2. Over use accessory muscles
3. Barrel chest
4. Diminished respiratory movements
5. Finger clubbing
6. Reduced exercise tolerance
   (cough/sputum not particular features)
   (termed 'pink puffers' − breathless but not cyanotic)

Complications
Respiratory failure (slow onset)
Corpulmonale

Principles of physiotherapy
1. Aid patient in best use of healthy lung tissue
2. Encourage efficient, controlled breathing
3. Encourage relaxation
4. Improve control/co-ordination of respiration during normal activity
5. Improve thoracic mobility/general exercise tolerance
6. Prevent respiratory infection − remove secretions
7. Assist patient to understand condition and role in treatment

Treatment methods
1. Local relaxation
2. Basal breathing control
3. Controlled breathing during simple activity
4. Postural control/correction
5. Coughing
6. IPPB (if severe)

PNEUMONIA

Acute inflammation of lung substance, commonly infective origin, associated with systemic symptoms
Two types:
1. Bronchopneumonia
2. Lobar pneumonia

Predisposing factors
1. Lowered resistance
2. Viral infections
3. Chronic airways obstruction
4. General anaesthesia

Pathological changes
1. Bronchopneumonia
   (i) Inflammatory changes scattered throughout lungs (chiefly basal zones) with local epithelial destruction
   (ii) Inflammatory exudate/pus is produced which fills affected alveoli→consolidation or blocks off smaller airways→atelectasis (or both)
   (iii) Resolution follows, but fibrous tissue replaces damaged epithelium
2. Lobar pneumonia
   (i) Inflammatory changes localized to airways of one or more lobes (often pleura also)
   (ii) Vasodilatation→inflammatory exudate/pus which fills alveoli/terminal airways→consolidation
   (iii) Leucocytes/macrophages soften solid exudate, fluid remaining − either reabsorbed or expectorated→resolution if complete lung→normal

Signs and symptoms
1. Fever − acute onset
2. Dyspnoea − worsens with consolidation
3. Reduced respiratory movements
4. Cyanosis − if widespread
5. Confused − if diffusion defects present
6. Cough − *lobar* − initially dry and painful, with resolution→rusty coloured purulent sputum
   Broncho − purulent from beginning

Principles of physiotherapy
Rest, chemotherapy, oxygen if required
Physiotherapy aims to:
1. Encourage expectoration
2. Regain expansion of areas involved
3. Encourage early ambulation to mobilize secretions
4. Maintain full use of healthy lung
5. Increase length of expiration (improve gaseous exchange)
6. Improve general exercise tolerance/thoracic mobility
7. Encourage postural awareness/correction

Treatment methods
1. Coughing, vibrations/shaking
2. Modified PD
3. Humidification
4. Breathing control/relaxed expiration in all areas
5. General mobility exercises
6. IPPB/suction − if severe

Complications
1. Respiratory failure
2. Right heart failure
3. Incomplete resolution

BRONCHIECTASIS

Chronic dilatation of one/several bronchi/bronchioles with retention of bronchial secretions and persistent infection in affected lobe/segment. Commonly involves lower lobes

Causes
Following an infectious disease – thick sputum plugs cause areas of collapse
Bronchial obstruction
Congenitally weak bronchi
Chronic respiratory infections→fibrosis

Pathological changes
1. Bronchi/bronchioles are totally obstructed
2. Air distal to block gradually absorbed→collapse of distal airways
3. Obstructive agent→inflammatory changes in adjacent zone
   Mucosa loses sensitivity, walls weaken→fibrosis
   Secretions collect – secondary infection occurs
4. Fibrosis occurs in collapsed areas – contraction follows, which produces dilatation of weakened airways immediately proximal to blockage
5. Secretions collect in dilatations – 'spill' into adjacent airways→spread of infection
6. Inspiratory suction forces, traction, the dilatations – condition worsens

Signs and symptoms
1. Chronic cough – copious purulent sputum
2. Respiratory movements diminished in affected area
3. Reduced vital capacity
4. Haemoptysis
5. Digital clubbing
6. Halitosis
7. Frequently thin/lethargic, postural defects
8. General condition variable e.g.:
   a. 'Ill' – toxic absorption
   b. Generally well except for repeated chest infections

Complications
1. From spreading infection/toxic absorption – emphysema, cerebral/lung abscess, septic emboli
2. Recurrent pneumonia
3. Massive haemoptysis

Principles of physiotherapy

If condition localized — surgery performed e.g. lobectomy
If generalized, disease controlled by antibiotics/physiotherapy

Medical treatment

Physiotherapy aims to:
1. Remove retained secretions
2. Prevent spread of infection
3. Maintain full function of healthy lung tissue
4. Improve vital capacity, increase respiratory excursion
5. Improve patient's general condition — posture, mobility, vitality
6. Teach self care of chest/respiratory hygiene
7. Encourage patient to lead a normal life, hobbies/sport

Treatment methods

1. Coughing — clapping, vibrations
2. Accurate PD, suitable for home and department
3. Breathing control — all areas
4. Strap exercises
5. General mobility/agility exercises

CORONARY HEART DISEASE

Causes

Predominantly a condition of high living standards — combined factors including obesity, smoking, hypertension, high blood cholesterol.

Myocardial infarct

Ischaemia to heart muscle affected→atrophy/necrosis. Fibrous tissue replaces necrosed area→'weak spot'. Results in reduced cardiac output/reserve, some degree of failure.

Principles of physiotherapy

1. Initially — complete rest/nursing care, relief from pain/shock oxygen/chemotherapy
   physiotherapy to prevent complications
2. Later — gradual mobilization within limitations, watch for signs of over-exertion, e.g. dyspnoea, tiredness, pallor, chest pain — if present stop treatment — rest
   Check pulse before/after exercise — rate should not rise more than 20 per minute and should be normal within 3 minutes
3. After 6–8 weeks — cardiac class, aimed to:
   (i) Strengthen cardiac muscle
   (ii) Increase cardiac output, improve reserve
   (iii) Reassure patient
   (iv) Increase endurance, mobilize/strengthen musculo-skeletal system
4. Give general advice — e.g. live within capabilities, take daily exercise, eat regularly but less fats, minimize mental strain

SURGICAL CHEST CONDITIONS

COMMON COMPLICATIONS OF THORACIC SURGERY

1. Lung collapse/consolidation
2. Cardiac arrythmia
3. CO_2 retention
4. Hypoxia
5. Circulatory complications − DVT, emboli
6. Surgical emphysema
7. Cardiac tamponade
8. Pleural effusion
9. Ventilatory/cardiac arrest
10. Restricted arm/trunk movements

Preoperative care

Investigations/tests
   (i)   Chest X-rays
   (ii) Sputum − culture/sensitivity, malignant cell count
   (iii) Blood tests − including gas analysis
   (iv) Dental examination − septic foci treated
   (v)   Respiratory function tests − thoracic excursion, vitalograph, peak
         flow; (vital capacity should be reasonable, if not surgery may
         create a 'respiratory cripple')
   (vi) Pulse rate, BP

Prior to lung surgery
   (i)   Bronchography if necessary
   (ii) Bronchoscopy to enable observation, biopsy, suction

Prior to heart surgery
   (i)   Electrocardiography − defects treated when possible, allows for
         post operative comparison
   (ii) Apex beat differential count − wide discrepancy indicates left
         sided malfunction (commonly left ventricular failure LVF)
   (iii) Cardiac catheterization − results detect degree of damage to
         each valve

Physiotherapy

PRE-OPERATIVE ASSESSMENT
History is taken and examination should include:
1. Shape of thorax
   Acquired/congenital deformity, influence post operative recovery
   NB (i)   Pectus carinatum/excavatium
   (ii) Barrel chest
   (iii) Kyphosis/scoliosis
   (iv) Assymmetry
2. Respiratory movements
   (i)   Amount in each area
   (ii) Symmetry in same area of opposing sides
3. Sputum — note type, quantity, viscosity
4. Indications of cardio-pulmonary insufficiency
   (i)   Cyanosis
   (ii) Digital clubbing
   (iii) Peripheral oedema
   (iv) Raised jugular venous pressure
   (v) Dyspnoea, orthpnoea, PND
5. Joint movement — note range in
   a.   Thoracic/cervical spine
   b.   Shoulder girdle/joints
6. Exercise tolerance
   Note speed/distance obtained — on the flat, up slopes/stairs
7. Cerebral function
   Note evidence of CVA cerebral insufficiency and generalized atherosclerosis
   Correlate results of objective tests/special investigations, estimate overall condition

Pre operative principles
1. Explain relevance and teach post operative procedures:
   (i)   Breathing exercises
   (ii) Coughing
   (iii) Postural awareness
   (iv) Arm, leg, general exercises
2. Encourage breathing awareness in all areas of thorax
3. Improve thoracic mobility by
   (i)   Trunk/shoulder girdle exercises
   (ii) Bilateral/unilateral rib movements
4. To remove secretions by:
   (i)   Coughing
   (ii) Modified PD
   (iii) Vibrations/shaking
   (iv) Inhalation therapy
5. Reassurance/basic explanation of patient's role in early and later post operative period. Explain possibility that patient may return to another ward for 12–24 hours — intensive care unit

Post operative principles
1. Encourage maximum inspiratory effort — expand all lung tissue
2. Prevent lung collapse/consolidation by removing secretions:
   (i) Coughing
   (ii) Efficient controlled breathing exercises
   (iii) Vibrations/shaking
   (iv) Modified PD
   (v) Suction
   (vi) Alteration in volume/speed of air flow
3. Prevent circulatory complications by:
   (i) General bed mobility
   (ii) Foot/lower limb movements
   (iii) Early ambulation
   (iv) Deep breathing
   A non extensible webbing bandage tied to foot of bed assists general mobility
4. To improve/maintain thoracic, spinal, shoulder girdle/joint mobility by:
   (i) Passive movements (if unconscious)
   (ii) Active assisted/active movement
   (iii) Resisted movement
   (iv) Postural awareness/correction
5. To enable patient to return to as full and active life as possible

Post operative assessment
On returning from theatre prior to treatment the physiotherapist should note:
   (i) Surgery undertaken — incision used
   (ii) Drainage tubes — number and position, type/quantity of drainage
   (iii) Other tubes present e.g. endotracheal, Ryles'
   (iv) BP, temperature, pulse rate
   (v) Respiration —
      a. Spontaneous — rate/depth
      b. Artificial — rate, pressure, volume
   (vi) ECG, blood gases
   (vii) X-ray — compare films
   (viii) Drugs — type, quantity, time of administration
If coincide, analgesics assist treatment

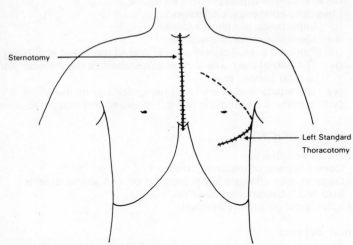

Fig. 3. Common Thoracic Incisions

Principles of physiotherapy when patient is on a ventilator

1. Chest care
   (i) To prevent infection by removing excess secretions
      – suction combined with shaking, vibrations, rib
      springing, manual hyperinflation (bagging)
   (ii) To prevent lung collapse/consolidation by altering
      rate/depth of respiration – achieved by regular (2 hourly)
      hyperinflation techniques/forced inflations
   (iii) To maintain/reduce viscosity of secretions – if tenacious,
      saline may be infused into airways

2. Movement and positioning
   Variable according to:
   (i) Reason for artificial ventilation
   (ii) Patient's general condition
   When appropriate the physiotherapist should
      a. Instruct patient to perform routine maintenance exercises
      b. Perform active assisted/free exercise to maintain joint
         range, muscle power/length, and aid venous return
      c. Perform passive movements to maintain joint range,
         muscle length and aid venous return (when patient
         paralysed/unconscious)
      d. Position the patient so good posture can be maintained

3. General care and preventative medicine
   Physiotherapist must understand:
   (i) Importance of charts/records
   (ii) Medical problems involved
   (iii) Patient's overall condition and amend treatment accordingly
   (iv) The role of the nurse and other members of the medical team in total patient care
   (v) The equipment in use, and recognize any malfunction
   (vi) Importance of regular turning to avoid pressure sores

VALVULAR LESIONS

May be acquired due to:
1. Complications of rheumatic fever
2. Degenerative changes superimposed on congenital defects
3. Sub acute bacterial edocarditis
Mitral valve most frequently involved.

Valvular defects
1. Stenosis – small orifice, difficulty in opening→back pressure
2. Incompetence – inadequate valve closure, reduced outflow of blood, regurgitation occurs→back pressure
3. Combination of 1. and 2.
   Surgery is either:
   (i) Valvotomy
   (ii) Valve replacement
   (iii) Annuloplasty

Pathological changes
Basically the same whichever valve is affected.
1. Cusps thick/rigid, with calcium deposits on valve margins
2. Chordae tendineae often short, thick and fused together

MITRAL VALVE

Stenosis (more common)

Effects
1. Left ventricle (LV) slightly smaller — less blood enters
2. Raised pressure left atrium (LA)→LA hypertrophy
3. Back pressure in pulmonary circulation
4. Pulmonary congestion/hypertension
5. Back pressure in right ventricle (RV) → RV
   hypertrophy→heart failure

Signs and symptoms
1. Pulmonary oedema
2. Dyspnoea — graded 1–4 according to severity
3. Orthopnoea, PND
4. Haemoptysis
5. Malar flush
6. Atrial fibrillation
7. X-ray changes

Incompetence

Effects
1. Ventricular systole→regurgitation LV→LA
2. Reduced cardiac output
3. LA pressure rises→increased LV filling on diastole (Starling's Law)
4. →LV hypertrophy→greater incompetence
   Eventually LVF
5. Increased LV filling→greater stroke volume, compensating for reduced cardiac output (BP maintained)
6. Raised LA pressure→pulmonary hypertension (less severe than stenosis)

Signs and symptoms
Early — tiredness, palpitations
Later — enlarged heart, displaced apex beat, exertional dyspnoea, orthopnoea
Much later — pulmonary congestion/oedema, ascites

AORTIC VALVE

Stenosis

Effects
1. Less blood in aorta
2. More blood in LV, pressure rises→LV hypertrophy
3. Reduced cardiac output→reduced coronary circulation
4. Insufficient blood for hypertrophied LV→LVF
5. LVF→raised pulmonary pressure

Signs and symptoms
None until LVF
1. Angina
2. Dyspnoea

Incompetence (more common)

Effects
Good compensation present, despite large reflux. Cardiac output —
normal at rest, slight rise on exercise.
Compensation for less blood in aorta achieved by:
1. Blood from LA/refluxed blood→raised LV pressure
2. LV stretched→stronger systole→increased stroke volume
   (cardiac output maintained)
3. Limit of LV hypertrophy reached→atrophy LV→LVF, aortic
   pressure falls
4. Coronary circulation reduced — insufficient for working
   muscle→increasing LVF

Signs and symptoms
None until LVF
1. Exertional dyspnoea, later dyspnoea at rest
2. Angina on effort, later continual pain

TRICUSPID VALVE

Stenosis

Effects
1. Reduced filling RV→small RV
2. More blood right atrium (RA)→RA hypertrophy
3. Back pressure→systemic venous congestion

Signs and symptoms
1. Hepatomegaly, ascites
2. Oedema – sacral, ankles
3. Raised jugular venous pressure

Incompetence

Effects
1. Blood to RA on RV systole, less enters lungs
2. Raised pressure RA, RA stretches→greater diastolic filling RV
3. RV stretches→greater incompetence

Signs and symptoms
As in stenosis but less severe

PULMONARY VALVE
Disorders almost always congenital

Stenosis

Effects
1. Resistance to blood flow→RV hypertrophy
2. Pulmonary circulation reduced
3. Less blood passes to LA/systemic circulation

Signs and symptoms
1. Fatigue
2. Exertional dyspnoea→dyspnoea at rest
3. No peripheral cyanosis at rest, may be on exertion

Incompetence
Almost always due to raised pulmonary pressure.
Back pressure to RV makes valve incompetent.
Signs of pulmonary congestion/systemic venous congestion.

CONGENITAL HEART DEFECTS

Possible causes
1. Defective/arrested development in early foetal life
2. Maternal rubella during pregnancy
3. Amniotic adhesions affecting growth symmetry
4. Genetic factors

Disorders may be divided into:
1. ACYANOTIC
   Characterized by:
   (i) No peripheral cyanosis
   (ii) No shunting of blood, or left→right shunting
2. CYANOTIC
   Characterized by:
   (i)   Peripheral cyanosis
   (ii) Shunting of blood right→left
   (iii) Increased pressure in right heart

Acyanotic conditions	*Cyanotic conditions*
Valvular stenosis	Tetralogy of Fallot
Atrial septal defect (ASD)	Transposition of great vessels
Ventricular septal defect (VSD)	
Persistent ductus arteriosus (PDA)	
Aortic co-arctation	

Each may occur separately or co-exist.

Common signs and symptoms
1. Acyanotic
   (i)   Child thin, small/slow development
   (ii) Exertional dyspnoea
   (iii) Recurrent respiratory infections
   (iv) Excessive fatigue/weakness
   (v)   Diarrhoea/vomiting
   (vi) Cyanotic/dyspnoeic attacks
2. Cyanotic
   (i)   Central cyanosis
   (ii)   Digital clubbing
   (iii) Polycythemia
   (iv)   Squatting position adopted
   (v)   RV hypertrophy
   (vi)   Fainting, dizziness – cerebral hypoxia
   (vii) Paraesthesia in extremities

In both
   (i) Heart murmurs
   (ii) Abnormal cardiac shadow

ASD
Foramen ovale remains patent
Blood passes LA→RA
Less blood enters aorta→decreased BP

VSD
Septal maldevelopment→left→right shunting
More blood passes to lungs/left heart→RV/LV hypertrophy

PDA
Ductus arteriosus remains patent
Oxygenated blood diverted from aorta→lungs
Peripheral blood volume/pressure decreased

TETRALOGY OF FALLOT
Combination of defects→
1.   RV hypertrophy
2.   Right→left shunt
3.   Less blood in lungs→reduced oxygenation
4.   Mixed blood in aorta
5.   Polycythemia

FURTHER READING:

Burton, J. L. (1973) *Aids to Undergraduate Medicine.* Edinburgh:
   Churchill Livingstone.
Burton, J. L. *Aids to Post Graduate Medicine.* Edinburgh:
   Churchill Livingstone.
Cash, J. E. *Chest, Heart and Vascular Disorders for Physiotherapists.*
   London: Faber & Faber.
Cole, R. B. (1971) *Essentials of Respiratory Disease.* London: Pitman.
Cumming, G. & Semple, S. J. (1973) *Disorders of the Respiratory
   System.* Oxford: Blackwell.
Owen, S. G., Stretten, T. B. & Vallance-Owen, J. (1969) *Essentials of
   Cardiology.* London: Lloyd Luke.

Obstetrics and gynaecology

COMPLICATIONS OF PREGNANCY AND THEIR PHYSIOTHERAPY TREATMENT

1. *Breathlessness and/or pulmonary disease*
   Breathing exercises, posture correction and relaxation.
2. *Cramp*
   Foot and leg exercises
3. *Oedema of the arms and legs*
   Exercises in elevation
4. *Round ligament pain/sacro iliac pain*
   Posture correction and relaxation
5. *Costal margin pain*
   Breathing exercises, posture correction and relaxation
6. *Backache*
   Localized, superficial heat, posture correction and relaxation
7. *Varicose veins*
   Foot and leg exercises
8. *Rheumatic, congenital and other heart diseases*
   Breathing exercises and relaxation

OTHER COMMON COMPLICATIONS OF PREGNANCY NOT TREATED BY PHYSIOTHERAPY

1. Abortion – threatened, inevitable, complete, incomplete, missed, recurrent or habitual
2. Ectopic pregnancy
3. Multiple pregnancy
4. Vomiting
5. Heartburn
6. Urgency of micturition and/or stress incontinence
7. Haemorrhoids
8. Cystitis
9. Incompetent cervix
10. Placenta praevia
11. Placental insufficiency
12. Anaemia
13. Pre-eclamptic toxaemia
14. Diabetes
15. Maternal physical abnormalities

ANTE NATAL TRAINING

Principles of physiotherapy
To give the pregnant woman the confidence she needs to be in control of her labour by:
1. Giving her a clear understanding of pregnancy and labour
2. Giving advice on posture control and correction
3. Teaching the patient the breathing patterns and relaxation techniques which will be of help during labour
4. Giving advice on the role of the husband in labour
5. Preparing her for the post-natal period

Methods of treatment
1. Classes held in the hospital where the patient is to be delivered
2. Classes held in Local Health Clinics
3. Psychoprophylaxis
4. Private tuition

POST NATAL TRAINING

Principles of physiotherapy
1. To correct posture
2. To restore the correct breathing patterns
3. To restore the tone in the abdominal and pelvic floor muscles
4. To stimulate the circulation

Methods of treatment
1. A clear verbal explanation is essential as the patients are not ill
2. Posture correction in all positions
3. Diaphragmatic and lateral costal breathing exercises
4. A progressive scheme of abdominal and pelvic floor exercises
5. Advice on lifting, etc.

LABOUR

Signs of labour
1. A 'show' of blood stained mucus
2. Ruptured membranes
3. Regular contractions

Stages of labour
1. The first stage is the time taken for the cervix to reach full dilatation. Contractions gradually get stronger and more frequent and some discomfort may be felt in the lumbar region.
2. The second stage is when the baby passes through the cervix and along the vaginal canal to the outside world. Strong contractions are supplemented by the efforts of the mother.
3. The third stage is the removal of the placenta which usually occurs a short time after the baby is born.
A lot of patients are helped in labour by the administration of an epidural anaesthetic during the first stage.

COMMON GYNAECOLOGICAL CONDITIONS TREATED BY PHYSIOTHERAPY

Prolapse, cystocele, rectocele

Signs and symptoms
1. Discomfort and heaviness in the vulval area
2. Backache
3. Frequency of micturition and/or stress incontinence
4. Occasional pain or burning on micturition

Stress incontinence

Signs and symptoms
1. Loss of urine on exertion
2. Frequency and/or urgency of micturition
3. Backache and/or low abdominal pain
4. Constipation

Causes of A and B
Loss of pelvic muscle tone due to:
1. Childbirth
2. Disease
3. Obesity
4. Senility

Principles of physiotherapy
1. To increase pelvic and abdominal muscle tone
2. To restore and increase voluntary pelvic floor control

Treatment
1. Pelvic floor and abdominal exercises, or
2. Pelvic floor faradism and exercises, or
3. Surgery followed by exercises

Pelvic inflammatory disease

Signs and symptoms
1. Diffuse abdominal pain sometimes with swelling
2. Increased vaginal discharge and irritation
3. Backache
4. Increased menstrual flow and dysmenorrhoea
5. Deep dyspareunia
6. Anaemia
7. General lethargy

Causes
1. Pelvic disease
2. Infection following surgery
3. Ruptured ectopic pregnancy or appendix
4. Endometriosis
5. Venereal disease

Principles of physiotherapy
1. To help reduce infection
2. To relieve pain

Treatment
1. Cross-fire short wave diathermy
2. Gentle mobilizing exercises
3. Relaxation

Dysmenorrhoea

Signs and symptoms
1. Pre-menstrual tension
2. Menstrual pain
3. Backache
4. Nausea
5. Vomiting
6. Fainting

Causes
1. Fear and misunderstanding of the menstrual cycle, i.e. tension
2. Pelvic inflammatory disease
3. Genital abnormality

Principles of physiotherapy
To reduce pain and tension

Treatment
1. Vigorous exercise to stimulate pelvic circulation
2. Short wave diathermy if infection is present
3. Relaxation
4. Dilatation and curettage

COMMON SURGICAL CONDITIONS TREATED
BY PHYSIOTHERAPY

Hysterectomy
1. Sub-total hysterectomy is the removal of the body of the uterus. It is rarely done because of the possibility of cancer of the cervix in later life.
2. Total hysterectomy is the removal of the uterus and cervix. It may be done in conjunction with a unilateral or bilateral salpingo-oophrectomy when there is disease of the tubes and ovaries.
3. Wertheim's hysterectomy is performed because of Stage II or III cancer of the cervix and uterus. It is the removal of the ovaries, fallopian tubes, uterus, cervix, upper half of the vagina, parametria and pelvic lymph glands.

Indications for hysterectomy
1. Cancer
2. Dis-functional bleeding
3. Inter-menstrual bleeding
4. Menorrhagia
5. Fibroids

Pelvic floor surgery
1. Pelvic floor repair is performed to correct varying degrees of prolapse.
2. Vaginal hysterectomy is done when there is a procidentia or when uterine disease complicates a lesser form of prolapse.

Indications for pelvic floor surgery
1. Severe stress incontinence
2. Prolapse

Radical vulvectomy
Radical vulvectomy is extensive surgery done for carcinoma of the vulva. It is a block dissection of the vulva, mons veneris, clitoris and perineal tissue. It often involves skin grafting.

Principles of physiotherapy
1. To maintain good respiratory function
2. To maintain circulation
3. To restore abdominal and pelvic floor muscle tone

Treatment
1. Pre and post operative localized breathing exercises and coughing
2. Exercises to maintain circulation
3. Exercises to restore abdominal and/or pelvic muscle tone
4. Posture correction

FURTHER READING:

Bourne, G. (1972) *Pregnancy*. London: Cassell.
Garland, M. D. & Quixley, J. M. E. (1971) *Obstetrics and Gynaecology for Nurses*. English University Press.
Heardman, H. (1959) *Physiotherapy in Obstetrics and Gynaecology*. Edinburgh: Churchill Livingstone.
Jenkins, D. ed. (1975) *Having a Baby*. Expectant Mothers Service.

Soft tissue injuries and sports medicine

The basic aims and means of treatment of recent trauma are the same no matter how the injury is caused. There are, however, certain factors to be considered when dealing with sports injuries.

1. Athletes are not average people
2. Complex psychological effect
3. Specialized rehabilitation
4. Different sports have typical injuries
5. Highly developed muscles waste quickly

ASSESSMENT OF INJURY is based on the same principles as those used by the medical officer see Adams (1972)

1. To decide aims and methods of treatment
2. To allow accurate recording of progress

Investigation as to occurrence
When? Where? How?
Pain. Region, type, time factors

Observation
Soft Tissues:
Contour. Swelling
Skin changes: Colour, texture, laceration, etc.
Bones and Joints: Position relative to anatomical normal

Detailed inspection and palpation
Skin: Temperature. Colour
Pulses
Muscles: Wasting, power, range, spasm, laceration
Tendons
Bones: Changes in position of prominences, depressions, local tenderness
Joints: Deformity. True or false movement. Active/passive range comparison.
Region of pain in both types of movement
Crepitus
Ligaments
Nerves: anaesthesia. parasthesia

Principles of physiotherapy
A tabulated list prepared at a Sports Clinic is ideal for reference.
See Steel (1972)
Important points:
1. Regain/maintain joint stability and mobility
2. Regain/maintain muscle function
3. Re-establish co-ordination
4. Maintain general fitness, including cardio-respiratory efficiency
5. Quick return to activity:
    (i) Not to the detriment of the patient
    (ii) Not achieved by the use of trick movements

Classification of injury
1. Bone as the primary site of injury (See fractures page 110)
2. Joint as the primary site of injury
3. Where bone and joint are not the primary site of injury
There may be a combination

JOINTS AS THE PRIMARY SITE OF INJURY

Structures in and around the joint are concerned with stability and mobility and the balance between the two

Degrees of displacement
Dislocation: articular surfaces completely displaced
Subluxation: partial separation beyond normal
Sprain: overstretch of a joint with ligamentous damage but the joint returns to normal position

Possible structures affected
Capsule. Capsular ligament. Synovial membrane
Ligaments. intra/extra capsular
Tendons and tendon sheaths
Bursae
Non-articular cartilage e.g. menisci
Amount and consistency of synovial fluid in the joint

Dislocation
Most commonly caused by long leverage, occasionally with shallow joints, by approximation of surrounding parts

Signs and symptoms
1. Tearing sensation
2. Intense pain easing to an ache
3. Abnormality of shape
4. Abnormal movement and/or limitation of movement
5. Muscle spasm
6. Loss of function

Pathological changes
Acute inflammation
Inflammatory exudate leading to possibility of fibrous adhesions
Muscle wasting may occur

Assessment
See page 98

Principles of physiotherapy
1. Reduction
2. Immobilization
3. Maintenance, where movement is permitted
4. Prevent adhesions
5. Early mobilization with weight or stress relieved and within limit
   of pain, but opinions differ
   Progress is made bearing in mind:
   (i) Direction of dislocation
   (ii) Particular precautions necessary for each joint
6. Re-education of functional movement

Possible techniques
1. Cold therapy
2. Immobilization:
   Sling for upper limb. Additional splintage if necessary
   Traction, splintage or bed rest for lower limb
3. Isometric exercises
4. Passive movement within pain free range
5. Assisted movement: must be well taught and supervised
6. Neuromuscular facilitation
7. Active movement with gradual progression
8. Resistance: springs and weights
9. Ultrasound. Short wave diathermy. Infra-red
10. Group therapy for functional activity once full range is obtained

Complications
1. Fractures
2. Periosteal involvement
3. Capsulitis
4. Synovitis
5. Injury to nerves. Stretch or compression
6. Injury to blood vessels
7. Ischaemia
8. Skin or subcutaneous tissue involvement
9. Limitation of range
10. Abnormal movement patterns
    Gravitational swelling may occur in the limb involved if
    preventative measures are not explained and implemented

Subluxation
The principles of treatment are the same but with immediate treatment and quicker progression.

Sprain
Similar but less severe signs and symptoms with occasionally a more localized pain. Ligament and capsular involvement are common.

Principles of physiotherapy
1. Immobilization
2. Reduce inflammation
3. Prevent/control swelling
4. Avoid muscle wasting
5. Avoid formation of fibrous adhesions
6. Maintain full range movement in joint and in surrounding areas
7. Obtain full functional activity

Frequently affected joints, knee, ankle, wrist

Knee
Philip Wiles suggests that with a minor sprain there should be only minimal modification of normal activity with avoidance of extra stress positions. Twisting, turning, quick starting and stopping, etc.
See Wiles & Sweetman (1965).
Activity should be maintained where possible to avoid atrophy of the quadriceps.

Important to examination
With a complete rupture of the medical ligament, the knee may appear stable in extension, therefore test in varying degrees of flexion.

Signs and symptoms
1. Pain – acute tenderness over injury site
2. Effusion depending on severity and position
3. Joint instability in severe cases. Tested according to function of ligaments involved
4. Local oedema
5. Inflammatory reaction
6. Difficulty with efficiency of extensor mechanism

Signs and symptoms for sprains in other regions, similar except 6

Possible techniques
1. Cold therapy
2. Compression
3. Elevation
4. Circulatory exercises in elevation as allowed by splintage
5. Immobilization.
   Compression bandage is often sufficient
   Splint or plaster of paris in severe cases
6. Isometric exercises for quadriceps
7. Flexion as soon as pain permits. Never forced
8. Ultrasound
9. Frictions. Although frictions produce good results in many cases, the upper attachment of medial ligament is an example of a situation where they may be contraindicated, the danger being Pellegrini – Steida's disease.

The close proximity of structures in and around the knee determines that if trauma occurs the injury sustained may be collective, e.g. O'Donaghue triad. See O'Donaghue, (1950).

Meniscus injuries
The medial meniscus is most commonly affected. In function of the knee an increase in pressure between femur and tibia and including the menisci occurs during extension. Increase beyond a functional degree produces a common sign of this injury, namely, 'locking'. Overlapping of fragments is usually responsible.

Signs and symptoms
1. Difficulty with full extension of knee
2. Joint occasionally 'locks' on slight flexion
3. Rotation is absent in last few degrees of extension
4. Pain at joint level
5. Traumatic synovitis
6. Clicking noise on movement

Complications
1. Limitation of range
2. Instability of joint
3. Muscle wasting or imbalance
4. Osteoarthrosis

Treatment
Surgical: meniscectomy
Follow-up physiotherapy according to the wishes of the surgeon
Time factor is variable

Comment
Personal preference is for early treatment, particularly when dealing
with athletes.
Isometric exercises and some straight leg raising from first
post-operative day. Flexion only commenced after removal of sutures.
Straight leg raising only works the quadriceps statically with the
exception of Rectus Femoris, and should occupy only a small part of
the exercise time.

*A guide for quick assessment with a view to progress to group
therapy in the gymnasium*
  1. No effusion
  2. 90° flexion
  3. No extensor lag
  4. Fairly strong quadriceps. Able to lift a small weight through full
     range extension
  5. Hospital transport not required
Only in extremely rare cases is electrotherapy required
In combined injuries the treatment of the ligament takes precedence

Ankle

Treatment
Early use of cold and compression
Severe cases — plaster of paris
Intermediate stage — contrast bathing
Maurice Ellis sets out a progressed treatment of adequate
immobilization associated with contrast bathing and progressive
exercises. See Ellis (1972)
The damaged ligament should be in a shortened position when
supported
Grade 1 Compression. Non stretch adhesive strapping applied over
gamgee tissue
Contrast bathing
Non weight bearing
Grade 2 Adhesive stretch strapping and felt pads over local sites
Commence weight bearing
Grade 3 Adhesive stretch strapping

Exercises
Early stage. Do not stretch affected ligaments
Progression — range, strength
A 'wobble board' is ideal for function

Wrist
Immediate use of cold therapy
Support by a metal, plastic or plaster of paris splint
Principles of treatment as with other sprains
The tendons and sheaths require additional consideration

Complications of sprains
1. Oedema
2. Synovitis
3. Periostitis
4. Chronic sprain
5. Osteoarthrosis

Synovitis
The synovial membrane is frequently involved in joint trauma. Continual overstretching, even slight, may result in an inflammatory reaction.

Signs and symptoms
In acute cases the changes are typical of any inflammatory reaction and can be seen after only a short time
1. Effusion
2. Fluctuating swelling
3. Joint sometimes red
4. Aching-type pain is predominant

Possible techniques
1. Cold therapy
2. Compression
3. Elevation
4. Isometric exercises
5. Circulatory exercises to other joints where possible
6. Progressive active exercise
7. Short wave diathermy is beneficial if a wider circulatory effect is required
8. Ultra sound given marginally

Teno synovitis
Caused by an irritant which is either internal or external to the membrane
1. Tearing of fibres of tendon or sheath
2. Repeated stress, even slight
3. Direct blow
4. Repeated pressure
The inflammation may lead to fibrous adhesions

Signs and symptoms
1. Pain particularly on movement, acute along the tendon involved
2. Swelling – more often localized
3. Aching in surrounding area
4. 'Grating' feeling on movement

Possible techniques
1. Cold therapy
2. Splintage
   Compression with orthopaedic felt pads and adhesive strapping
   may be sufficient
3. Ultra sound
4. Short wave diathermy for late developing pain/swelling
5. Frictions after the acute stage
6. Passive stretching
7. Heat treatment for relaxation and circulatory effect
   Some people suggest faradism at the later stage if re-education of
   individual muscles is required. This is not often necessary but has
   proved valuable in some cases.

Tennis elbow
Opinions vary as to exact definition. See Adams (1971) and
Wiles and Sweetman (1965)

Examples of lesions
Lateral ligament strain
Capsular involvement
Bursitis in the common extensor tendon
Overstretch of fibres of Extensor Carpi Radialis longus or brevis, usually
at the musculo-tendinous junction

Cause
Strong forearm movement, particularly involving pronation and
supination associated with strong gripping is commonly responsible.
Rugby players, golfers, engineers are common sufferers, possibly more
so than tennis players.

Signs and symptoms
1. Pain emphasized on forearm movement or pressure
2. Local tenderness
3. Muscle spasm
4. Localized pain but one complication in severe cases is aching and
   tension of arm and shoulder region

Principles of physiotherapy
Obtain and maintain full range movement. Pain on movement is likely to
persist until range is full.

Possible techniques
Listed by Joan E. Cash (1966) according to actual structure involved
1. Early stage — cold therapy
2. Supportive sling
3. Ultrasound
4. Short wave diathermy
5. Repeated stretching or manipulation, often in conjunction with an injection of local anaesthetic and hydrocortisone
6. Frictions
7. Heat for more extensive muscle spasm or widespread aching
8. Relaxation
9. Movement — Full range must be obtained quickly and then maintained because the tendency to heal in a shortened position may lead to a chronic condition

LESIONS WHERE THE BONE AND JOINT ARE NOT THE PRIMARY SITE OF INJURY
Tearing of muscle tissue
Contusion
Bursitis

Tearing of fibres of a muscle
Common injury in sport
May be situated:
1. In muscle belly
2. At musculo-tendinous junction
3. There may be periosteal involvement

Cases of spontaneous trauma frequently occur. Continuous overstrain may be the cause in athletes involved in heavy training programmes. Muscles passing over two joints are frequently affected.

Signs and symptoms
1. Pain, particularly on movement
2. Loss of power
3. Loss of stretch. In conditions where the facial planes between muscles are affected rather than the fibres, stretch may still show a good range
4. Muscle spasm
5. Aching
6. Swelling
7. Haematoma formation may be obvious

Principles of physiotherapy
1. Prevention or reduction of scar tissue
2. Maintenance of muscle length, flexibility and strength. In severe cases of muscle rupture, surgery may be indicated

Possible techniques
During first 24 hours:
1. Cold therapy
2. Compression. More rigid splinting is sometimes required
3. Elevation
   Athletes sometimes feel, particularly with intermuscular lesions, that they can 'run it off'. This is not true and will only aggravate the situation
   Massage is *contraindicated* and is a common mistake at sporting events
4. After the initial 48 hours, depending on severity, gentle stretching of the muscle is essential. See Gordon (1975)
5. Ultrasound
6. Short wave diathermy

Complications
1. Scar tissue/fibrous formation which limit muscle function
2. Myositis ossificans. Common site, quadriceps
3. Further tearing of surrounding tissue
4. Atrophy of damaged or sometimes adjacent muscles
5. Periostitis where damage occurs close to bony attachments

Contusion
A heavy blow is the cause and muscle tissue is crushed
Bleeding may be quite extensive
Common sites: Thigh, gluteal region

Signs and symptoms
1. Affected part hard and swollen
2. Haematoma may be obvious after only a short time depending on the severity of the force involved
3. Restricted movement
4. Painful movement
5. Inflammation
6. Spasm in surrounding muscles

Principles of physiotherapy
1. Dispersion of haematoma with minimal scar formation
2. To maintain flexibility, elasticity and strength of the muscle

Possible techniques
1. Cold therapy
2. Compression. In lower thigh lesions compression should include the knee to avoid gravitational swelling into the joint
3. Elevation
4. Isometric exercises
5. Circulatory exercises to limb
6. Ultrasound
7. Short wave diathermy. Indirect application for wider circulatory problems
   Directly given to site only after haematoma is more isolated
8. Progressive exercises within pain limit
9. Gentle stretching after the inflammatory reaction has subsided
10. Modified massage at later stages

Bursitis

Bursitis is included in this section because injuries affecting the deeper bursae are usually part of a more complicated disturbance already mentioned. The more isolated types of bursitis are those which are obvious because of their superficial position.

Cause
A direct heavy blow
Repeated less severe blows
Continual pressure
Prepatellar and olecranon bursitis are common particularly in body contact sports and in miners

Signs and symptoms
1. Swelling usually localized
2. Pain on pressure
3. Pain on any movement which increases pressure on the walls of the envelope of membrane

Principles of physiotherapy
Dispersion of the fluid whilst maintaining normal range is important as the initial inflammatory reaction subsides

Possible techniques
1. Cold therapy if seen at time of injury
2. Rest and support
3. Ultrasound
4. Localized short wave diathermy
5. Progressive exercise within limit of pain and which does not put pressure on the bursa
6. Chronic stage. Massage including marginal frictions
7. Surgical removal may be necessary

This brief outline includes only some techniques particularly in the later stages. First aid measures for all soft tissue injuries should include:
1. Application of cold
   The exception to this is external bleeding, which must be controlled before any further treatment
2. Compression to provide support

The most important factor is the use of exercise. Electrotherapy may help. The co-operation of all concerned is essential but not always easy to achieve, especially in sport.

FURTHER READING

Adams, I. D. (1972) The management of the injured sportsman. *Physiotherapy*, **58**, 6–200.

Adams, J. C. (1971) *Outline of Orthopaedics*. London: Churchill Livingstone.

Cash, J. E. ed. (1966) *Physiotherapy in Some Surgical Conditions*. London: Faber & Faber.

Ellis, M. (1972) *Casualty Officers Handbook*. London: Butterworth.

Gordon, H. M. (1975) Physiotherapy in muscle strains of the lower limb. *Physiotherapy*, **61**, 4, 102.

O'Donaghue, D. H. (1950) The surgical treatment of fresh injuries to the major ligaments of the knee. *Journal of Bone and Joint Surgery*, **32A**, 721.

Steele, V. (1976) St. James' Hospital Sports Clinic. *Physiotherapy*, **62**, 8, 246.

Wiles, P. & Sweetman, R. (1965) *Essentials of Orthopaedics*. London: Churchill.

Fractures and orthopaedics

Fractures are discontinuity of bone structure caused by trauma or pathology

CLASSIFICATION
Through normal bone
1. Closed. Skin intact
2. Open (compound). Skin damaged

Fractures may be solitary or multiple

Through abnormal bone
Pathological

CAUSES
Traumatic
1. Direct force. Soft tissue damage
2. Indirect force
   Rotational – spiral
   Angulatory – transverse
   Compression – often a separate bony fragment
3. Muscular force
   Avulsion of muscle attachment to bone
4. Stress fracture

In cancellous bone, direct force results in a crush fracture

Pathological
(Force applied insufficient to break normal bone)
1. Congenital
   (i)   Osteogenesis imperfecta
   (ii) Osteopetrosis
2. Infective
   (i)   Pyogenic osteomyelitis
   (ii) Syphilis
3. Metabolic
   (i)   Osteoporosis
   (ii) Osteomalacia
4. Dysplasias
   (i)   Paget's disease
   (ii) Simple cyst
   (iii) Fibrous dysplasia

General complications
1. Venous thrombosis, pulmonary embolism
2. Fat embolism
3. Crush syndrome

HEALING OF FRACTURES

Tubular bone (compact)
Haematoma
Subperiosteal and endosteal cellular proliferation
Callus formation − soft woven bone
Consolidation of woven bone to compact bone
Remodelling to normal shape

Cancellous bone
Haematoma
Penetration by blood vessels
Proliferation of osteogenic cells from fractured surface
Action of osteoblasts
Formation of intercellular matrix
Calcification

Factors influencing healing of bone
1. Quality of fixation
2. Closeness of coaptation after reduction
3. Age
4. State of bone and underlying disorder
5. Extent of injury
6. Infection
7. Inadequate blood supply
8. Interposition of soft tissue between fragments
9. Dissolution of haematoma by synovial fluid
5. Tumours
   (i)   Secondary
   (ii) Myeloma
   (iii) Primary

SYMPTOMS

1. Pain
2. Loss of function

SIGNS

Local
1. Swelling and haemorrhage
2. Deformity
3. Tenderness
4. Abnormal movement
5. Crepitus

General
1. Shock
2. Other injuries
3. Evidence for pathological fracture

RADIOGRAPHS (two views)

Reveal:
1. The exact site
2. Pattern of fracture
3. Degree and direction of displacement

PATTERN OF FRACTURES

1. Transverse
2. Oblique
3. Spiral
4. Comminuted
5. Compression or crush
6. Greenstick

DISPLACEMENT

1. Tilt or angulation
2. Rotational
3. Overlap
4. Shift
5. Impaction

COMPLICATIONS

1. Local
2. General

Local complications

Bone
1. Delayed union. Union taking longer than expected, but may still occur
2. Non union. Union will not occur spontaneously
3. Mal union. Bone unites in a deformed position
4. Avascular necrosis. Death of bone following damage to the arterial blood supply
5. Infection

Joints
1. Adhesions from oedema and immobilization
2. Mal union may limit joint range
3. Myositis ossificans. Deposition of calcium around joints
4. Sudeck's atrophy. Cause unknown. Pain and stiffness
5. Late traumatic arthritis

Muscle and tendon
1. Tearing of muscle fibres and tendons
2. Avulsion of tendon attachment to bone
3. Post traumatic tendonitis
4. Muscle wasting

Nerve
1. Neuropraxia. Most common
2. Axonotmesis. Where there has been traction
3. Neurotmesis. Rare in closed fractures

Artery
Arterial blood supply may be impaired in both open and closed fractures
1. Disruption of a major vessel
2. Thrombosis
3. Intimal damage
4. Compression by tissue. Pressure from oedema, bleeding, tight plaster

Features of impaired arterial perfusion
1. Pain
2. Pallor
3. Paraesthesia
4. Pulselessness
5. Paralysis
Complete obstruction of arterial flow for several hours results in gangrene
If obstruction is incomplete, or transient, severe damage to nerves and muscles may result, e.g. Volkmann's ischaemic contracture

Skin
1. Primary damage
   (i) Contusion, laceration, crushing and skin loss degloving
2. Secondary damage
   (ii) Fracture blisters, plaster sores, bed sores

Viscera
1. Brain and spinal cord
2. Abdominal organs
3. Thoracic viscera

General complications
1. Venous thrombosis, pulmonary embolism
2. Fat embolism
3. Crush syndrome

TREATMENT OF FRACTURES

Principles of treatment
   First aid and reduction
   Immobilization
   Restoration/preservation of function

Reduction
1. Closed
2. Open. Indications
   (i) Where closed treatment fails
   (ii) When accurate reduction is obligatory

Immobilization – aims to:
1. Prevent malunion
2. Limit risk of non union
3. To relieve pain

Methods of immobilization

Plaster of paris/Thomas' splint
Immobilization of adjacent joints
Prevents rotation by immobilizing both the joint above and below the fracture

Continuous traction
1. By gravity
2. Skin traction
3. Skeletal traction
4. Fixed/static or
5. Balanced/dynamic

Internal fixation
Using metal implants
1. Intramedullary fixation
2. Fixation by plates screws nails and pins

Indications for internal fixation
Absolute
1. Pathological fractures of long bones
2. Where two major long bones in the same limb are fractured
3. Where there is injury to nerves or major vessels

PHYSIOTHERAPY IN TREATMENT OF FRACTURES

Principles of physiotherapy
1. Maintain normal movement and function of non injured structures
2. Restore normal movement and function as soon as possible of fractured area

Assessment is necessary before and during treatments
1. Record relevant information
2. Read notes and radiographs
3. Discuss with surgeon and ward sister
4. Understand splintage and surgical treatment

Note the following:
1. Cause of fracture
2. Other injuries or illnesses
3. Complications
4. Occupation
5. Home situation

Examination
Ask patient about their symptoms
1. Pain
2. Stiffness
3. Function

Look for
1. Changes in colour
2. Skin changes
3. Oedema
4. Effusion
5. Muscle wasting

Feel for
1. Tenderness
2. Local heat

Test
1. Muscle action
2. Joint range
3. Sensation
4. Respiratory function
5. Functional activities

PRINCIPLES OF PHYSIOTHERAPY

Co-operation with other members of team
1. Surgeon
2. Nurse
3. Occupational Therapist
4. Social Worker
5. Resettlement Officer
6. Family

Explanation and instruction to patient
1. Explain aims of treatment whenever possible:
   (i)   Joint range to be achieved
   (ii) Muscle power to be regained
   (iii) Function to be restored
2. Teach exercises to be practised
   (i)   State frequency
3. Teach functional activities to be practised

Reduce oedema
1. Exercises in elevation
2. Deep breathing exercises to assist venous return
3. Support for dependent limb

Maintain respiratory function for patients with:
1. History of respiratory disease
2. Injury of thoracic cage
3. Spinal injury
4. Weak or paralysed intercostal and abdominal muscles

Reduce pain of soft tissue by:
1. Ice
2. Ultrasound
3. Heat
4. Movement

Period of immobilization
1. Maintain full movement of all joints not splinted
2. Exercise all muscles – isometrically where no movement is allowed
3. Encourage functional activities and independence

Period of mobilization
Re-education of movement
1. Mobilize still joints
2. Strengthen muscles
3. Restore equilibrium
4. Retrain independence

Suggested techniques – re-education of movement
1. To mobilize joints
   (i)   Free exercise
   (ii) Hydrotherapy
   (iii) PNF hold or contract relax
   (iv) Suspension therapy
   (v)   Passive mobilization
2. To strengthen muscle
   (i)   PNF straight resistance
   (ii) Repeated contractions
   (iii) Pulleys and weights
   (iv) Spring resistance
   (v)   Use of body weight

PHYSIOTHERAPY FOR PATIENTS WITH FRACTURES OF THE UPPER LIMB

Independence activities to be encouraged when in plaster and during period of mobilization:
1. Feeding
2. Writing
3. Dressing
4. Toilet
5. Household duties (waterproof covering of plaster for activities involving water)

Exercises for patients to practise when in plaster:
Performed in elevation in the presence of oedema

Hand
1. Flexion and extension of fingers
2. Full flexion of metacarpal phalangeal joints must be maintained
3. Adduction and abduction of fingers
4. Flexion and extension of thumb
5. Opposition of thumb

Shoulder
1. Elevation
2. Adduction in flexion
3. Abduction in flexion
4. Extension
5. Rotation

Elbow
Flexion and extension

Treatment after removal of splintage:
Advice to patient:
1. Care of the skin
2. Position of the limb for comfort, especially at night
3. Position of the limb to overcome oedema
4. Activities to be performed
5. Exercises to practise

To overcome pain and discomfort:
1. Ice
2. Wax
3. Movement in water
4. Infra-red radiation

Techniques to re-educate movement:
1. Exercises combining movements of all joints and muscles
   (i) PNF patterns
   (ii) Hydrotherapy
2. Movements localized to individual joints
   (i) Free
   (ii) Assisted
   (iii) Passive mobilization where joint stiffness persists
3. Resistance exercises to weak muscle groups using:
   (i) Gravity
   (ii) Manually (PNF)
   (iii) Pulleys and weights
   (iv) Springs
   NB No resistance should be given distal to fracture until fracture is solid
4. Retrain all grips:
   (i) Pincer
   (ii) Light
   (iii) Heavy

PHYSIOTHERAPY FOR PATIENTS WITH FRACTURES OF THE LOWER LIMB

Patient's immobilized in bed

Maintain extensor tone and prevent flexion contracture of hip and knee
1. Lie flat for definite period each day, prone if possible
2. Isometric exercises for gluteal and quadriceps muscles
3. Active exercises for non injured and injured leg (if permitted)

Maintain full movement of foot and ankle
1. Adequate foot support for patients on traction, especially for the elderly
2. Active exercises of all movements foot and ankle, particularly for dorsi-flexors of the ankle and flexors of the toe

Maintain good circulation in the leg
1. Vigorous plantar flexion exercises of foot
2. Active exercises of non injured leg
3. Deep breathing exercises

Check splintage is in correct position and does not impede permitted movement
1. Knee flexion piece of Thomas splint
2. Plasters to allow full hip, knee and toe movement (if below knee plaster)

Treatment when splintage removed: patient not ambulant
See techniques for re-education of movement upper limb

Exercises for mobilization of lower limb could include:
1. Hydrotherapy
2. Free and assisted movement in all planes
Simple suspension, abduction and adduction of hip (ropes suspended from monkey pole)
Sliding board, abduction and adduction hip
Knee:
Wedge on pillow under thigh: extension of knee
Spring resistance, knee extension (spring suspended from monkey chain)
Prone, flexion and extension of knee
Foot and ankle:
Crook lying, knees to right and left alternately for eversion and inversion foot
Spring resistance to plantar flexion (spring suspended from monkey pole)

Treatment when patients are ambulant

Training in independence activities, such as:
1. In and out of bed
2. Standing to sitting in chair
3. Dressing
4. Toilet
5. Gait training
6. Steps
7. In and out of car
8. On and off bus

Activities in preparation for return to work e.g.
1. Climbing (bricklayer)
2. Balancing (bricklayer, bus conductor)
3. Lifting (lorry driver)
4. Bending (gardener, housewife)

Gait training
1. Elasticated support in presence of oedema
2. Commence training in pool or parallel bars

Weight bearing depending on union of fracture
1. Non weight bearing (NWB) on axillary crutches
2. Partial weight bearing (PWB) on axillary/elbow crutches
3. Full weight bearing (WB) gradually discard aid

Progress re-education of movement
1. Exercises to strengthen muscle and mobilize joints. (No resistance distal to fracture until solid)
2. Pulleys and weight in PNF patterns
3. Spring resistance
4. PNF straight resistance. Repeated contractions
5. Body weight resistance
6. Passive mobilization techniques where stiffness persists

Balance and equilibrium
1. Various weight bearing exercises
2. Use of wobbly board
3. Progress to circuit training

CRUSH INJURIES OF THE HAND

Cause of injury
1. Mostly industrial
2. Heavy machinery
3. Road traffic accidents

Tissues injured can be:
1. Skin
2. Blood vessels
3. Nerves
4. Muscles and tendons
5. Bones
6. Joints

Signs and symptoms
1. Swelling
2. Pain
3. Stiffness
4. Motor and sensory loss
5. Loss of function

Immediate treatment
1. Cleaning and debridement of wound without tourniquet
2. Primary repair of nerve and tendons if wound is clean
3. Reduction and fixation of fractures
4. Repair of skin by suture, graft or flap
5. Application of compression bandage
6. Hand in safe position
7. Arm elevated

Later surgery
1. Reconstruction of finger or thumb
2. Tendon graft
3. Nerve repair
4. Skin graft

Principles of physiotherapy
Preservation of movement is vital
Oedema must be reduced

Immediate treatment
1. Active movements all joints in elevation
2. Encourage functional activities

Treatment when bandages are removed
1. Full active movements. Movements can be enhanced by use of:
    (i)   Silicone oil
    (ii) Ultrasound
    (iii) Wax
    (iv) Ice
2. Grip training
3. Progressive strengthening exercises of all muscles of upper limb
4. Functional activities
5. Training for home and work

CRUSH INJURIES OF THE CHEST

Frequently associated with other injuries

Causes of injury
1. Road traffic accidents
2. Industrial injuries

Injuries may include:

Bone
1. Ribs
    (i)   Usually multiple
    (ii) More than one fracture in each rib
    (iii) Fracture most common at angle of ribs and usually fifth to ninth rib
2. Sternum
3. Spine
4. Clavicle

Soft tissue injuries
1. Lung – puncture wounds or crushing
2. Pleura
3. Trachea or bronchus – rupture
4. Intrathoracic vessels – usually fatal
5. Oesophagus
6. Pericardium
7. Heart – usually fatal

Complications leading to respiratory embarrassment or failure include
1. Flail (stove in) chest which may result in paradoxical breathing
2. Imploding chest (from fractured sternum and clavicle)
3. Airway obstruction
4. Collection of secretions
5. Lung collapse
6. Pneumothorax – often with surgical emphysema
7. Haemothorax
8. Pain

Immediate treatment aims to
1. Maintain clear airway
2. Maintain respiratory efficiency

Clearance of secretions by one of the following
1. Naso tracheal aspiration
2. Endo tracheal tube
3. Tracheostomy
4. Physiotherapy. Modified postural drainage, chest shaking, breathing exercises
5. Inhalations (tinc benz)

Maintenance of adequate ventilation by the use of
1. Intermittent positive pressure ventilation
2. Positive and expiratory pressure
3. Physiotherapy — as above

Management of pain
1. Analgesia — respiratory depressants avoided
2. Local anaesthesia
   (i)   Locally into site of rib fracture
   (ii) Regionally by intercostal nerve block
   (iii) Regionally by epidural block
3. Entonox inhalation
4. Intermittent positive pressure ventilation

Rarely are the following operations carried out for fractured ribs
1. Rib traction as an emergency procedure with towel clips
2. Wire suture
3. Intra medullary pin fixation
4. Introduction Rush nails
5. Pin fixation sometimes to stabilize chest wall

INJURIES OF THE SPINE

Structures which could be injured
1. Spinal column
   (i) Fractures
   (ii) Dislocations
2. Spinal cord/nerve roots
3. Lung, pleura
4. Abdominal viscera
5. Pelvic viscera

Fractured spine

Types of fracture
1. With or without dislocation
2. Compression wedge fracture of vertebral body
3. Burst fracture of vertebral body

Cause of fracture
Trauma
1. Falls from height giving fracture of lumbar spine. Can be associated with fracture calcaneum
2. Direct force at site of fracture
3. Crush injury
4. Force from above: Flexion and rotational force to cervical spine
5. Whiplash injury: Flexion followed by hyperextension to cervical spine
Pathological
1. Osteoporosis
2. Tumour

Treatment of spinal fractures
There are two overriding considerations:
1. Is the fracture stable or unstable?
2. Is there neurological damage?

Where the fracture is stable
Rest in bed initially and when pain settles external splintage, collar, corset or plaster
Early mobilization

Displaced and unstable fractures
Traction to obtain and hold reduction (for cervical spine Crutchfield Calipers)
Open reduction and fixation with plate and screws

Physiotherapy for patients on traction or bed rest (where there is no cord involvement)

Cervical spine fractures
1. Movements of legs and lumbar spine
2. Movements of arms but care in elevation to avoid moving cervical spine
3. Isometric contractions of gluteal and quadriceps muscles
4. Deep breathing exercises

Dorsal spine
1. Movements of arms and legs
2. Deep breathing exercises

Lumbar spine
1. Movements of arms
2. Single leg movement
3. Isometric exercises gluteal and quadriceps muscles

Progression when surgeon permits to:
1. Prone, extension exercises
2. Gradually mobilization exercises and ambulation
3. Progressive strengthening exercises of all muscle groups
4. Training in lifting
5. Posture training

Spinal cord lesions
Can be a complete or partial transection
Resulting in:
1. Paralysis
   (i)   Tetraplegia at cervical levels
   (ii) Paraplegia at lower levels
   Can be flaccid or spastic depending on site of lesion
2. Sensory loss (deep and superficial)
3. Incontinence (bowel and bladder)
4. Loss of vaso-motor response, and
5. Sexual function – impotence in the male

Early complications of cord injury
1. General and spinal shock
2. Pain
3. DVT
4. Pulmonary embolism
5. Respiratory failure in high lesions

Complications of paralysis
1. Respiratory impairment (paralysis of intercostals and abdominals)
2. Contractures which are painful
3. Immobility
4. Loss of independence

Other complications
1. Pressure sores
2. Respiratory infection
3. Urinary tract infection
4. Peri articular ossification – especially of shoulder and hip
5. Depression

Early treatment of spinal cord lesions
1. Introduction of bowel and bladder management
2. Tracheostomy and ventilation for patients with high lesions and respiratory impairment
3. Good bed posture and regular change of position to
   (i)   Prevent contractures
   (ii) Minimize spasticity
   (iii) Prevent pressure sores
4. Application of splints in prevent contractures
   Feet supported at 90° with padded foot board
   Metacarpal joints splinted at 90° flexion with inter phalangeal joints extended and thumb in opposition

Physiotherapy for the acute lesion

Assessment is essential before treatment
Examination of the following:
1. Muscles noting
   (i)   Spasticity
   (ii)   Flaccidity
   (iii) Muscle imbalance
   (iv)   Reflex responses
   (v)   Muscle shortening
   (vi)   Contractures
2. Joints noting
   (i)   Range
   (ii)   Contractures
3. Respiratory function
   (i)   Test vital capacity
   (ii)   Observe intercostal diaphragmatic and abdominal movement and action of accessory breathing muscles
   (iii) Examine for secretions in the lungs

Treatment
1. Respiratory physiotherapy
2. Passive movements
3. Facilitation of movement as recovery is observed

Physiotherapy for the early ambulant patient. (Adapted to each patient according to level of cord lesion)

Re-education of movement
1. Inhibitory techniques for muscle spasm
2. Facilitation of muscle action
3. Strengthening muscle

Training in independence
1. Sitting up and lying down
2. Turning over in bed
3. Balance in sitting
4. Dressing
5. Washing
6. Feeding

Training in self care
1. To prevent pressure sores and trauma to skin
2. Methods of relieving pressure

Progression of treatment

Re-education of movement
1. Progressive resistance exercises
2. Mat work
3. Hydrotherapy

Training in independence
1. Transfers to and from wheelchair, car, lavatory, bed, etc.
2. Wheelchair activities
3. Standing from wheelchair
4. Balance in standing
5. Application of caliper
6. Gait training

Training in self care
Bladder and bowel training

Training in preparation for home
1. Involvement of the family in rehabilitation
2. Home visits for short periods initially
3. The Occupational Therapist will assess and recommend adaptations to home and supply appropriate aids

AMPUTATIONS

Amputation is the ablation of the whole or part of a limb

Amputation may be:
1. Traumatic
2. Surgical

Surgical amputation is undertaken for the following reasons
1. To save the patient's life (crush syndrome, tumour)
2. To prevent the spread of infection (gas gangrene)
3. To improve mobility and function (gross deformity)

Conditions which may necessitate amputation of the limbs
1. Peripheral vascular disease (often diabetic patients)
2. Gross and multiple injuries
3. Malignant bone disease — osteosarcoma
4. Infection — gas gangrene, osteomyelitis
5. Gross deformity
6. Flail limb (brachial plexus lesion of the upper limb)

Levels of amputation

Lower limb
1. Hind quarter
2. Disarticulation of the hip
3. Mid thigh — most common in elderly with vascular disease
4. Through knee or Gritti Stokes (retaining the patella)
5. Below knee
6. Syme's
7. Toes

Upper limb
1. Forequarter
2. Disarticulation of shoulder
3. Upper arm amputation
4. Mid fore arm
5. Fingers or thumb

Post operative management (depending on site of amputation)
1. Wound is drained for two to three days
2. Patient is allowed up after two or three days
3. Application of stump bandage applied
4. Immediate prosthesis applied in few days (lower limb)
5. Permanent prosthesis fitted later

Principles of pre-operative physiotherapy
1. Gain the patient's confidence
2. Assure respiratory function
3. Commence the rehabilitation programme by teaching appropriate exercises

Principles of post operative physiotherapy

Prevention of contractures
1. Posture and positioning of stump
2. Appropriate exercises

Control oedema
1. Exercises for all muscle groups of stump
2. Stump bandage
3. Regular wearing of prosthesis

Strengthen muscles of:
1. Stump
2. Trunk (for double amputees)
3. Arms (for crutch walking)
4. Scapular (for upper limb amputee)

Functional training
Application and care of prosthesis
Lower limb
1. Mobility
2. Dressing
3. Toilet
Upper limb
1. Training in use of prosthesis usually undertaken by Occupational Therapists in special units
2. Preparation for home and work

CORRECTIVE BONE AND JOINT SURGERY

Indications
  1. Disabling pain
  2. Instability
  3. Deformity

Types of corrective operations

Osteotomy
(i)   Bone divided close to joint
(ii)   Deformity corrected by excision of wedge
(iii) Internal/external fixation applied

Arthrodesis
(i)   Surgical fusion of a joint
(ii)   Bone graft or metal fixation used

Excision arthroplasty: Complete excision of joint

Interposition arthroplasty: Prosthesis placed between joint surfaces

Partial arthroplasty. Articular surface or part of joint replaced

Total arthroplasty.

Operation	Site	Post Operative Management
Osteotomy	Upper femoral	Hip movements in a few days Patient up when wound healed Partial weight bearing until osteotomy united
	Upper tibial	No external splintage Gradual mobilization in two to three days. Weight bearing almost immediately
	Double osteotomy (upper tibia lower femur)	Plaster cylinder. Gradual weight bearing in few days. Plaster removed about five weeks. Mobilize. Probably require manipulation under general anaesthesia
Arthrodesis	Hip	No external splint. Mobilize other joints. Non weight bearing gait when wound healed. Weight bearing when bony union
	Knee	Plaster cylinder until joint fused
Excision arthroplasty	Hip	Traction about three weeks, hip and knee movements. Mobilize in bed further three weeks. Then partial weight Foot and ankle movements. Walk on heel in few days. Movements all joints when stitches out. Gait training
	First toe (MP joint) Kellar's or Mayo's	
Interposition arthroplasty	Hip (cup)	Bed rest three to four weeks Partial weight bearing two weeks
Partial joint replacement	Hip (Thompson's)	Patient mobilized in few days. Full weight bearing
	Knee tibial plateau (Mackintosh)	Compression bandage five days then mobilize. Partial weight bearing
Total joint replacement	Hip Charnley	Abduction pillow one week. Assisted movement in two days. Ambulate about seven days
	McKee-Farrar	Assisted movements immediately. Ambulate about five days
	Knee Freeman (unrestrained)	Plaster two to three weeks or compression bandage then mobilize
	Stanmore (hinge type)	Plaster back slab about two weeks then mobilize

Physiotherapy
Important to understand
1. Nature of operation
2. The available range of prosthesis
3. The surgeon's wishes for post operative management

Treatment includes
1. Isometric exercises for major muscle groups
2. Movement of all other joints
3. Lying flat to prevent contractures of hip and knee
4. Progression to mobilizing and strengthening exercises
5. Gait training
6. Check leg length. Adjust shoe accordingly
7. Functional training

SPINAL SURGERY
1. Laminectomy
2. Fusion
3. Decompression

LAMINECTOMY

Indications
Prolapsed intervertebral discs where:
1. Symptoms are not relieved by conservative methods
2. Neurological signs, i.e. bladder complications
3. Acute pain and neurological signs (emergency treatment)

Types of operative procedure
1. Partial laminectomy
2. Fenestration. (Interlaminar approach)
3. Total laminectomy plus fusion

Post operative treatment
1. Horizontal bed rest for one week
2. Gradual mobilization
3. Discharged two to three weeks

Physiotherapy
Assess for neurological change throughout post operative treatment

First week
1. Patient horizontal from three days to one week
2. Breathing exercises
3. Isometric exercise of main muscle groups
4. Leg exercises including straight leg raise
5. Rolling from side to side
6. Prone lying about five days, active extension exercises
7. Patient up five to seven days

Second week onwards
1. Gradual mobilizing exercise including hydrotherapy
2. Progressive exercises for trunk muscles
3. Gradual sitting when stitches removed
4. Instruction in back care

SPINAL FUSION

Surgical fusion of two or more vertebral joints using bone graft or metal plate and screws

Indications
Unstable spine due to
1. Paralysis
2. Fractures/dislocations
3. Following laminectomy
4. Spondylolisthesis

Internal splintage to promote healing for
1. Tuberculosis
2. Fractures/dislocation

Post operative treatment
Patient horizontal three to four weeks
No movements of spine allowed
Up about four weeks wearing support

Physiotherapy
Breathing and leg exercises
Gradual ambulation
Function training

DECOMPRESSION

Removal of laminae and any other structures compressing the cord or nerve roots

Indications
Spinal stenosis
Nerve root compression intervertebral foramina
Compression by tumour

Post operative treatment
As for laminectomy

SOFT TISSUE RELEASE

Indications
1. Contractures
2. Loss of mobility
3. Pain

Types of operation
1. Tendons: Tenotomy
2. Capsule: Capsulotomy
3. Fascia: Fasciotomy

Post operative management
Full stretch of tissue maintained till tissue healed
Possible splintage

Physiotherapy
Exercises to maintain the increased range
Passive stretching in some instances

TENDON REPAIR

TYPES OF SURGERY

Transfer
Tendon of a strong muscle released from bone attachment reinserted on to a bone or into another tendon. Used to supplement or substitute for the action of a paralysed or weak muscle

Graft
A length of tendon (e.g. palmaris longus, plantaris) divided from donor muscle and sutured to recipient tendon or tendon and bone to:
1. Make up for loss of tendon substance
2. Lengthen a tendon
3. Replace a damaged tendon which has become scarred or adherent

Postoperative treatment
Elevation
Light splintage or compression bandage
Limb in position to avoid overstretch of repaired tendon
Gentle mobilization

Physiotherapy

Pre-operative physiotherapy
Mobilize the joint(s) over which the tendon will work
Strengthen all muscles of limb
Active exercise of all limb
Explain post-operative treatment

Post-operative physiotherapy
Exercise limb in elevation
Active exercise for all joints not splinted
Splintage removed (always observe carefully activity of repaired tendon):
  1. Active exercise all joints
  2. DO NOT PUT TENDONS ON FULL STRETCH TILL SURGEON SAYS SO
  3. Flex one joint whilst extending the other
For tendon transplant:
  1. Train muscle in its new function
  2. Encourage normal active movements
  3. Functional training
  4. Grip training

DEFORMITIES

Classification
  1. Congenital or acquired
  2. Postural or structural

Congenital deformities

Causes
  1. Genetic factor
  2. Factors in maternal environment:
     (i)   Nutrition
     (ii) Infection
     (iii) X-ray irradiation
     (iv) Chemical (drugs, i.e. thalidomide)
     (v)   Posture of foetus (i.e. foot deformity)
  3. Idiopathic
  4. Trauma at birth, e.g. fractures, Erb's palsy of arm

CONGENITAL DEFORMITY	DESCRIPTION OF DEFORMITY
CONGENITAL DISLOCATION OF HIP (CDH)	Dysplasia of acetabulum and femoral head Dislocation of femoral head up and backwards (Eight diagnostic signs) early diagnosis essential
FOOT DEFORMITIES 1. TALIPES EQUINO VARUS	As name implies
2. TALIPES CANEO VALGUS	As name implies
3. METATARSUS VARUS	As name implies
4. CONVEX PES VALGUS (VERTICAL TALUS)	As name implies
CONGENITAL TORTCOLLIS	Rotation of head to one side Lateral flexion to other side Unilateral contraction of sterno mastoid

SPINA BIFIDA	Three types:
	    1. Meningocele
	    2. Myelomeningocele
	    3. Spina bifida occulta
	Also other associated deformities, i.e.
	dislocated hip
	hydrocephalus, paraplegia

TREATMENT	SURGERY
Reduction by manipulation. Position maintained by splintage	1. After one year old Open reduction with removal of inverted lumbus 2. When deformity is established De-rotation osteotomy Salter osteotomy of pelvis Shelf operation Acetabuloplasty 3. In latter life Total hip replacement Arthrodesis
Manipulation and splintage to hold overcorrected position	For uncorrected or relapsed feet 1. Soft tissue release 2. Wedge resection of calcanum and cuboid 3. Calcaneum wedge osdeotomy 4. Tendon transplant 5. Arthrodesis
May correct spontaneously	Soft tissue release
Manipulation Splintage	Tendon transfer Ostectomy
Manipulation Stretching of sterno-mastoid Posture correction	Tenotomy of sterno mastoid
Management of paraplegia	Repair of lesion Corrective surgery to hips knees feet & spine
Cerebro-spinal fluid shunting (Spitz-Holter valve)	

ACQUIRED DEFORMITIES

Postural
No change in tissue
Can be corrected by patient's effort

Structural
Structural change in tissue
Cannot be corrected by patient's effort

Causes
1. Weak musculature
2. Debilitating illness
3. Persistent faulty posture

4. Secondary to another deformity, i.e. short leg leading to scoliosis

Causes
1. Muscle imbalance (paralysis)
2. Bony anomalies (Hemi — — vertebra)
3. Bone or joint disease, i.e. ankylosing spondylitis, Paget's disease
4. Bone growth disorders Scheuermann's disease

5. Idiopathic

DEFORMITIES OF THE SPINE

Deformity
Scoliosis: Curvature to one side

Treatment
Splintage:
   (i)   Milwaukee jacket
   (ii) Plaster jacket — Abbott or Risser
   (iii) Halo-pelvic traction
Surgery
   (i)   Fusion

Kyphosis: Exaggeration of dorsal curve
Lordosis: Exaggeration of lumbar curve. Nearly always postural or secondary to Kyphosis

Mainly treatment of underlying cause
Physiotherapy

DEFORMITIES OF LOWER LIMB

Mostly structural

Hip	*Treatment*
Flexion contracture	— Soft tissue release/splintage/manipulation
Coxa vara	— Osteotomy

Knee	
Genu valgus	— Osteotomy
Genu varus	— Osteotomy
Genu recuvartum	— Caliper or possibly osteotomy

Foot	
Pes planus — many causes	— Depending on cause
Drop foot	— Drop foot splintage
	Physiotherapy
Spasmodic flat foot	— Plaster cast up to three months
Metatarsalgia	— Metatarsal bar or pad
	Physiotherapy

Toes	
Hallux valgus	— Kellar's or Mayo's operation
Hallux rigidus	— Rockered sole. Kellar's or Mayo's operation or arthrodesis
Hammer toe	— Excision and arthrodesis

GROWTH AND EPIPHYSEAL DISORDERS
(OSTEOCHONDRITIS)

Cause — vascular disturbance, ischoemia, trauma

Signs and symptoms — pain, limitation of movement, muscle wasting, limp, (lower limb)

Lesions	Treatment	Surgery
Perthes' — upper femoral	Splintage to preserve congruity of femoral head in acetabulum	Triplanar osteotomy of femur to replace head in acetabulum
Osgood Schlatter — tibial tubercle	Rest until symptoms settle. Possible splintage, e.g. plaster	
Kohler — tarsal navicular	Rest until symptoms settle Possible splintage, e.g. plaster	
Freiberg — second metatarsal	Rest until symptoms settle. Possible splintage, e.g. plaster	
Sever's — calcaneum	Rest until symptoms settle. Possible splintage, e.g. plaster	
Scheuermann's — vertebrae bodies	Rest until symptoms settle. Possible splintage, e.g. plaster	
Keinboch — carpal lunate	Rest until symptoms settle. Possible splintage, e.g. plaster	
Osteochondritis dissicans knee joint	Rest until symptoms settle Possible splintage, e.g. plaster	Fixation or excision of loose body
Slipped upper femoral epiphysis (associated with Frohlick's syndrome)		1. Knowles pins to hold position. Osteotomy of femur when epiphysis fused 2. Denis Dunn operation

SOME BONE DISORDERS

Osteomalcia	Osteoporosis	Paget's disease
Bone atrophy or rickets of elderly. Deficient absorption of calcium	Often idiopathic. Can occur after immobilization, steriod treatment, Sudeck's atrophy and other disorders	Osteitis deformans. Slowly progressive Cause unknown
	Common in the elderly. Pathological fractures easily occur	
Patient unwell. Generalized aching. Muscles weak and tender May have deformities	Symptom free Minimal deformity	Deformities, particularly long bones of upper limb Complications include cardiac failure and sarcoma.
Treatment: Vitamin D (Calciferol) Calcium	Treatment: Calcium, phosphorus and protein Physical activity	Treatment: Calcitonin

FURTHER READING: FRACTURES

Anderson, M. E. (1972) Physiotherapeutic management of patients on continuous traction. *Physiotherapy*, **18**, 51.

Apley, A. Graham (1973) *A System of Orthopaedics and Fractures*. London: Butterworths.

Owen, Robert (1972) Indication and contra indication for limb traction. *Physiotherapy*, **18**, 44.

Powell, Mary (1972) Application of limb traction and nursing management. *Physiotherapy*, **18**, 46.

Watson, Jones (1976) *Fractures and Joint Injuries*. Edinburgh: Churchill Livingstone.

FURTHER READING: CRUSH INJURIES OF THE HAND

Boyes, J. H. (1970) *Bunnell's Surgery of the Hand*. 5th edn. Philadelphia: J. B. Lippincott.

Gifford, D. (1974) Silicone oil for hand trauma. *Physiotherapy*, **60**, 350.

James, J. I. P. (1970) The assessment and management of the injured hand. *Journal of British Society for Surgery to the Hand*, **1**.

Wyn-Parry, C. B. (1976) *Rehabilitation of the Hand*. London: Butterworths.

FURTHER READING: CRUSH INJURIES OF THE CHEST

Gaskell, D. V. & Webb, B. A. (1974) *The Brompton Hospital Guide to Chest Physiotherapy*. London: Blackwell Scientific Publications.

Keen, G. (1975) *Chest Injuries*. Bristol: J. Wright.

Seal, P. V. (1974) Analgesia in the treatment of chest injuries. *Physiotherapy*, **60**, 134.

Watson, Jones (1976) *Fractures and Joint Injuries*, Vol. I. 166. Edinburgh: Churchill Livingstone.

FURTHER READING: INJURIES OF THE SPINE

Bromley, Ida (1976) *Tetraplegic and Paraplegia. A guide for Physiotherapists*. Edinburgh: Churchill Livingstone.

Guttman, Sir Ludwig (1973) *Spinal Cord Injuries. Comprehensive Management and Research*. London: Blackwell.

McCay, E., Hollings, E. M. & Nichols, P. J. R. (1969) Problems of living on wheels. A synopsis. *Physiotherapy*, **55**, 447.

FURTHER READING: AMPUTATION

Clarke-Williams, M. J. (1969) The elderly amputee. *Physiotherapy*, **55**, 368.

Crossland, S. A. (1974) Rehabilitation of the below knee amputee using the pre-formed socket. *Physiotherapy*, **60**, 50.

Davies, B. (1973) The lower limb amputee. *Physiotherapy*, **59**, 350.

Lucy, D. (1972) A temporary exercises prosthesis for use following amputation of lower limb. *Physiotherapy*, **58**, 67.

May, D. R. W. & Davis, B. (1974) Gait and the lower limb amputee. *Physiotherapy*, **60**, 166.

Moncur, S. D. (1969) The practical aspect of balance relating to amputees. *Physiotherapy*, **55**, 409.

Murdoch, G. (1969) Balance in the amputee. *Physiotherapy*, **55**, 405.

Verstappen, H. M. Ch. Thursing, C. M. & Mulder, W. J. M. (1972) A new development in powered prosthesis for the upper limb. *Physiotherapy*, **58**, 232.

FURTHER READING: CORRECTIVE BONE AND JOINT SURGERY

Apley, A. G. (1973) *A System of Orthopaedics and Fractures*. London: Butterworth

Benjamin, A. (1969) Double osteotomy for the painful knee in rheumatoid arthritis and osteoarthritis. *Journal of Bone and Joint Surgery*, **513**, 694.

Britain, H. A. & Howard, R. D. C. (1950) Arthrodesis. *Journal of Bone and Joint Surgery*, **32B**, 282.

Cash, J. (1976) *A Textbook of Medical Conditions for Physiotherapists*. London: Faber & Faber.

Charnley, J. (1960) Arthrodesis of knee. *Clinical Orthopaedics*, **18**, 37.

Charnley, J. (1967) Total prosthetic replacement of the hip. *Physiotherapy*, **53**, 40.

Freeman, M. A. R. F., Swanson, S. A. U. S. & Todd, R. C. (1973) Total replacement of the knee using the Freeman Swanson knee prosthesis. *Clinical Orthopaedics*, **94**, 153.

Jackson, J. B. Waugh, W. G. & Green J. P. (1969) High tibial osteology for osteoarthritis of the knee. *Journal of Bone and Joint Surgery*, **51b** 1, 88.

McIntosh, D. L. (1972) The use of hemiarthroplasty prosthesis for advanced osteoarthritis and rheumatoid arthritis of knee. *Journal of Bone and Joint Surgery*, **54B**, 244.

Newman, P. H. (1973) Surgical treatment for de-rangement of the lumbar spine. *Journal Bone and Joint Surgery*, **55B**, 7.

Schatzker, J. & Pennel, G. F. Spinal stenosis. A cause of canda equina compression. *Journal Bone and Joint Surgery*, **50B**, 606.

FURTHER READING: TENDON REPAIR

Boyes, J. H. (1970) *Bunnell's Surgery of the Hand*. Philadelphia: J. B. Lippincott Co.

Wynn Parry, C. B. (1976) *Rehabilitation of the Hand.* London: Butterworths.

FURTHER READING: DEFORMITIES

Cane, Fenella (1969) Walking training of the young child with myelomeningocele. *Physiotherapy*, **55**, 3.22.
Eckstein, H. B. (1977) Spina bifida. The overall problem. *Physiotherapy*, **63**, 182.
Gaskell, D. V. (1974) Physiotherapy for scoliotic patients in respiratory failure. *Physiotherapy*, **60**, 71.
James, J. I. P. (1967) *Scoliosis*. Edinburgh: Livingstone.
Kapila, Jeela (1977) Primary treatment of spina bifida. *Physiotherapy*, **63**, 184.
Kennedy, J. M. (1974) *Orthopaedic Splints and Appliances*. London: Ballière.
Manning, C. W. (1967–68) Surgical background to Scoliosis. *Journal of the Royal College of Physicians*, **2**, 77.
Manning, C. W. (1974) Scoliosis. *Physiotherapy*, **60**, 9.
Madden, B. K. (1977) Orthopaedic aspects of Spina Bifida. *Physiotherapy*, **63**, 186.
Powell, M. (1976) *Orthopaedic Nursing*. London: Churchill Livingstone.
Sharrad, W. J. W., Zachary, R. B., Lorber, J. & Bruce, A. M. (1963) A controlled trial of immediate and delayed closure of spina bifida cyctica. *Archives of Diseases in Childhood*, **36**, 16.
Sharrad, W. J. W. (1964) Posterior ilio psoas transplantation in the treatment of paralytic dislocation of the hip in children with myelomeningocele. *Journal of Bone and Joint Surgery*, **46B**, 426.
Sharrad, W. J. W. (1971) *Paediatric Orthopaedics and Fractures*. Edinburgh: Blackwell Scientific Publications.
Taylor, J. F., Oyemade, G. A. & Shaw, E. (1976) Primary treatment of rigid congenital T.E.V. *Physiotherapy*, **62**, 89.
Walton, A. (1969) Treatment of the infant and young child with myelomeningocele. *Physiotherapy*, **55**, 315.

FURTHER READING: GROWTH AND EPIPHYSEAL DISORDERS

Adley, A. Graham (1976) *A System of Orthopaedics and Fractures*. London: Butterworth.
Barry, Hugh, C. (1969) *Paget's Disease of Bone*. Edinburgh: Livingstone.
Duthie, R. B. & Ferguson, A. B. (1973) *Mercer's Orthopaedic Surgery*. London: Edward Arnold.

Diseases and injuries of the nervous system

HEAD INJURIES

Severity depends on degree of brain damage sustained, not on the extent of the skull fracture

Common causes
1. Road traffic accidents
2. Industrial accidents
3. Domestic accidents

Males more commonly involved than females, with the highest incidence in the 15–34 age group.

Brain injury results from:
1. Deceleration force – e.g. when the head is suddenly stopped by the dashboard in a road traffic accident
2. Acceleration force – e.g. knock out blow
3. Depressed fracture or penetrating wound of skull

Primary brain damage
1. Focal – with contusion or laceration at:-
   (i) Site of blow
   (ii) Site opposite blow ('contre-coup' injury)
2. Diffuse generalized: with neuronal damage and white matter shearing. The severity of this varies between minimal and extreme, and can be classified by:
   (i) Duration of coma
   (ii) Length of post traumatic amnesia

The term 'concussion' has previously been used for mild forms of this.

Secondary brain damage
May arise from:
1. Intra cranial haematoma
   (i) Extra dural haematoma
   (ii) Sub dural haematoma
   (iii) Intra cerebral haematoma
2. Cerebral oedema or swelling
3. Hypoxia from:
   (i) Damaged respiratory centre
   (ii) Direct trauma to lungs and thorax
   (iii) Hypotension – blood loss
   (iv) Depressant drugs – e.g. morphia

Mechanism of brain damage from hypoxia

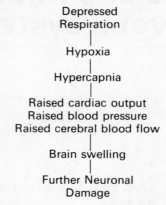

Depressed
Respiration
|
Hypoxia
|
Hypercapnia
|
Raised cardiac output
Raised blood pressure
Raised cerebral blood flow
|
Brain swelling
|
Further Neuronal
Damage

Prognosis

Factors influencing prognosis:
1. Degree of brain damage
2. Age of patient
3. Presence of thoracic trauma

Recovery following severe head injury is a gradual process and no clear division of stages may be made with any accuracy. However, the following categorization may provide a practical outline:
1. Unconscious stage
2. Sub conscious stage
3. Conscious stage

Principles of management of head injuries

To save life
1. Establish airway and adequate ventilation
    Respiratory depression or the presence of additional thoracic
    trauma may necessitate the use of any of the following:
    (i)   Endotracheal tube
          a. To provide unobstructed airway
          b. To facilitate suction
    (ii) Tracheostomy
          a. Necessary if the need for (i)a. and (i)b. extends beyond
              that of around 5–6 days
          b. To reduce dead air space
          c. To facilitate application of mechanical ventilation
    (iii) Intermittent positive pressure ventilation
          a. To increase respiratory function
    In all cases, any gas administered to the patient must be warmed
    and humidified. All precautions against sepsis must be taken.
2. Treat hypovolaemia and any additional trauma
3. Establish adequate recordings:
    (i)   Vital centres
    (ii) Neurological state
    (iii) Additional trauma
4. Control temperature

To minimise the sequelae of the injury
1. Establish general nursing routine:
    (i)   Skin
    (ii) Bladder and bowels
2. Provide adequate fluids and nourishment
3. Maintain full joint range of movement

Unconscious stage

Principles of physiotherapy
1. Assist in maintenance of free airway and adequate ventilation by:
   (i) Postural drainage within any limitations
        imposed by trauma and cerebral condition
   (ii) Vibration and rib springing
   (iii) Use of mechanical suction
   (iv) Bag squeezing
2. Inhibit development of abnormal patterns of reflex activity by:
   (i) Positioning to produce reflex inhibition
3. Maintain joint range and muscle length by:
   (i) Passive movements

Subconscious stage

Signs and symptoms — some or all of the following may be seen:
1. Increasing consciousness
2. Restlessness, irritation or confusion
3. Exaggerated response to stimuli
4. Return of cough and swallowing reflexes
5. Some voluntary movement

Principles of physiotherapy
No list may be given, since there is wide variation in clinical states
encountered. They may be seen as an extension of the principles of
treatment of the unconscious stage.

Conscious stage

Signs and symptoms — vary with the severity and the site of brain
damage. Any neurological dysfunction may be seen.

Assessment — see page 154

Principles of physiotherapy
1. Maintain airway and adequate ventilation by:
   (i) Breathing exercises
   (ii) Postural drainage
   (iii) Encouraging active coughing
2. Maintain joint range and muscle length by:
   (i) Passive movements
   (ii) Assisted and active movement
3. Inhibit abnormal patterns of reflex activity by:
   (i) Positioning to produce reflex inhibition
   (ii) Reflex inhibiting movement patterns
4. Establish communication
5. Increase sensory stimulus by:
   (i) Encouraging awareness of surroundings
   (ii) Afferent cutaneous stimuli
   (iii) Encouraging motivation
6. Develop normal tone
7. Develop balance reactions } by:
   (i) Functional movement in a developmental sequence
   (ii) Weight transference techniques
   (iii) Facilitation of isolated joint movement in a proximal-distal sequence
   (iv) Development of the ability to place the limb in space
8. Facilitate voluntary movement
9. Re-educate functional activities by:
   (i) Choice and adaptation of activities which do not conflict with other principles of treatment
   (ii) Choice and use of aids

Common complications following head injury
1. Post traumatic epilepsy – i.e. developing more than one week after injury – affects five per cent of all head injuries
2. Myositis ossificans – deposits of bone found in muscles and joint structures (Ectopic calcification) may be associated with:
   (i) Presence of long bone fractures
   (ii) Vigorous stretching of hypertonic muscles
3. Neuro-psychological disorders – e.g.
   (i) Behavioural changes
   (ii) Memory and learning deficits

MULTIPLE SCLEROSIS

Disease of unknown aetiology characterised clinically by a wide variety of signs and symptoms and pathologically by patchy demyelination of the brain and spinal cord.

Distribution
More common in cold and temperate climates; initial attack frequently between 20–45 years

Disease pattern
Classically, the pattern is of exacerbation and remission. Overall picture is of a progressive disorder with an unpredictable time scale. The average duration of the disease is 20 years.

Infective illness, trauma, surgery or pregnancy may be followed by an exacerbation.

Pathology
In areas up to 1 cm in diameter of brain and spinal cord:
1. Inflammation
2. Infiltration of leucocytes and plasma cells
3. Degeneration of myelin
4. Reactive gliosis
5. Sclerosis

Signs and symptoms
Relate to the site of the pathology and any combination of signs and symptoms may co-exist.
1. Motor:
   (i) Hyper-reflexia
   (ii) Weakness
   (iii) Spasticity — initially extensor, later flexor
2. Visual:
   (i) Retrobulbar neuritis — giving symptoms of
       a. Blurring of vision which may progress to uniocular blindness
       b. Pain on eye movements
   (ii) Diplopia
3. Psychological:
   (i) Euphoria
   (ii) Depression
4. Cerebellar:
   (i) Nystagmus
   (ii) Tremor
   (iii) Ataxia
   (iv) Alteration of postural tone
   (v) Dysarthria
5. Sensory:
   (i) Paraesthesiae
   (ii) Proprioceptive loss
6. Urinary:
   (i) Frequency
   (ii) Hesitancy
   (iii) Incontinence

Medical treatment
No specific therapy, but steriods often given in exacerbations.
Symptomatic therapy as listed, may be indicated for
1. Bladder symptoms
    (i)   Infections – antibiotics
    (ii) Dysfunction – bladder neck surgery
                        anticholinergic drugs
2. Respiratory infection – antibiotics
3. Muscle spasm – antispasmodics
                    phenol injections
                    orthopaedic surgery
4. Depression – anti-depressant drugs

Assessment – see page 154

Principles of physiotherapy
1. Maintain mobility and promote function by:
    (i)   Advice on sleeping postures, sitting postures, working
          positions
    (ii) Instruction in gait patterns
    (iii) Advice on choice and use of aids and appliances
    (iv) Provision of home exercise programmes
2. Minimize effects of exacerbations
    Specific programmes to treat dominant symptoms – see page 00
    NB Several symptoms may co-exist and treatment programmes
    must therefore be designed to avoid conflicting aims

HEMIPLEGIA

Disorder of movement of one side of the body arising from damage
to the brain or upper segments of the spinal cord.

Common causes
A. Cerebrovascular disease
B. Space occupying lesions
C. Trauma

Cerebrovascular disease
1. Infarction
    (i)   Thrombosis
    (ii) Embolus
          a. from heart – e.g.
             myocardial infarction; fibrillation
          b. from atheromatous plaques in other vessels
    Infarction accounts for over 60 per cent of all hemiplegia

Contributing factors
1. Disease of vessels – atheroma, arteritis
2. Diseases of blood – anaemia, polycythaemia
3. Disorders of blood flow – reduced cardiac output, e.g. syncope,
    myocardial infarction, arrhythmia

Common sites
1. Internal carotid artery
2. Middle cerebral artery
3. Anterior cerebral artery
4. Posterior cerebral artery

Onset
Develops over minutes or hours; not generally associated with activity and may occur during sleep.
Infarction — obstructs the blood supply to the area of the brain producing ischaemia and anoxia distally and consequently neurological damage.
2. Haemorrhage
    (i)   From normal vessels
          a. hypertension
    (ii) From abnormal vessels
          a. Aneurysm
          b. Angioma

Common site
Middle cerebral artery

Onset
Sudden with severe headache leading rapidly to loss of consciousness. May be associated with emotion or strenuous activity. Haemorrhage at the site of the lesion causes compression and disruption of brain tissue.

Space occupying lesions
1. Tumour
2. Abscess

Trauma — see page 145
Symptoms of residual hemiplegia may be found in any lesion affecting the motor cortex or internal capsule
Degree of damage depends on:
1. Severity of lesion
2. Site of lesion
3. State of collateral circulation

Signs and symptoms
Any or all of the following may be found:
1. Altered level of consciousness
2. Disturbance in communication
3. Disturbance in postural tone
4. Loss of voluntary movement
5. Sensory dysfunction
6. Visual disturbance
7. Intellectual impairment
8. Perceptual disorders
9. Incontinence

Assessment – see page 154
Hemiplegia occurs more commonly in the middle aged and elderly and therefore assessment of co-existing patholgy may also be necessary.

Principles of physiotherapy
1. Maintain airway and ensure adequate ventilation by:
    (i)   Breathing exercises
    (ii) Postural drainage
    (iii) Vibration
    (iv) Assisted coughing
2. Inhibit development of abnormal patterns of reflex activity by:
    (i)   Positioning to produce reflex inhibition
    (ii) Reflex inhibiting movement patterns
3. Establish communication
4. Increase sensory stimulus by:
    (i)   Weight bearing through limbs
    (ii) Afferent cutaneous stimuli
5. Maintain joint range and muscle length by:
    (i)   Passive movement
    (ii) Assisted active movement
6. Develop normal tone   (i)   Functional movement in
                                            a developmental
                                            sequence
                                     (ii)   Weight transference
                                            techniques
7. Develop balance reactions by: (iii) Development of isolated
                                            joint movement in a
                                            proximal to distal
                                            sequence
                                     (iv)   Development of the
                                            ability to place the limb
                                            in space
8. Facilitate voluntary movement   (v)   Use of afferent
                                            cutaneous stimuli
9. Re-educate functional activities by:
    the choice and adaptation of activities of daily living
    living in order that they do not conflict with other principles
    of treatment

Common complications
Painful shoulder
Oedematous hand
Persistent instability of ankle

ASSESSMENT OF CENTRAL NERVOUS SYSTEM

Mental
1. Consciousness
2. Orientation
3. Mood
4. Memory, attention span

Communication
1. Receptive ability
2. Expressive ability

Sensory
1. Cutaneous
   (i) Light touch
   (ii) Pressure
   (iii) Temperature
   (iv) Localization
2. Proprioception
3. Vision
   (i) Homonymous hemianopia
   (ii) Diplopia
   (iii) Nystagmus
4. Auditory
5. Perception
   (i) Execution
   (ii) Recognition

Motor
1. Passive
   - (i) Resistance to passive movement
   - (ii) Response to passive stretch
   - (iii) Range of painfree movement
2. Involuntary
   - (i) Tremor
   - (ii) Intention tremor
   - (iii) Abnormal reactions on attempted movement
3. Voluntary
   - (i) Isolated joint movement
     - a. Freely
     - b. From an inhibited position
   - (ii) Ability to support limb
     - a. Against gravity
     - b. In different parts of range
4. Balance
   - (i) Sitting
   - (ii) Kneeling
   - (iii) Standing
5. Weight transfer
   - (i) Rolling
   - (ii) Sitting
     - a. At hips
     - b. At arms
   - (iii) Kneeling
   - (iv) High kneeling
   - (v) Standing

Functional
1. Swallowing
2. Incontinence
3. Self care
   - (i) Feeding
   - (ii) Washing
   - (iii) Dressing
4. Movement in bed
5. Movement − bed to chair
6. Ambulation
   - (i) Flat ground
   - (ii) Rough ground
   - (iii) Stairs

Social
1. Family
2. Housing
3. Occupation
4. Way of life

Notes

Dysphasia/aphasia – loss of comprehension or of expression of spoken or written symbols of language

Dysarthria – paresis of muscles of articulation

Apraxia – inability to execute purposeful movement in the absence of motor paralysis, ataxia, sensory loss or deficiency of understanding

Agnosia – inability to recognize a familiar stimulus in the absence of a sensory deficit. May be:
1. Visual
2. Auditory
3. Tactile

Disorders of body image
1. Unilateral neglect – failure to use or acknowledge one side of the body
2. Anosognosia – lack of awareness or denial of disability

SYMPTOMATIC TREATMENT

The clinical picture which results from disease or damage to the central nervous system may show a dominant symptom or a combination of symptoms. Although symptoms are considered individually, it must be stressed that the effect of a specific technique must be observed on the whole patient. Assessment and treatment plans must be closely related.

Two common symptoms are:

SPASTICITY

State of hyper-tonicity of muscle characterized by:
1. An increase in sensitivity of stretch receptors, and
2. A release from cortical control of tonic reflex activity

Pain, pyrexia or joint contracture may induce an increase in spasticity.

Principles of physiotherapy
1. Inhibition of abnormal reflex activity by:
   (i)   Positioning to produce reflex inhibition
   (ii) Reflex inhibiting movement patterns
2. Facilitation of normal movement patterns by:
   (i)   Weight transference techniques
   (ii) Functional mat work with emphasis on rotation
   (iii) Functional movement in a developmental sequence
3. Decrease sensitivity of stretch reflex by:
   (i)   Cold therapy

ATAXIA

Disturbance of movement characterized by
1. Deficiency in postural tone
2. Loss of ability to coordinate movement

Principals of physiotherapy

1. Develop postural tone
2. Increase balance reactions
3. Develop coordinated movement
4. Re-educate functional activities

⎫ by: ⎬

(i) Stabilization techniques
(ii) Proprioceptive neuromuscular facilitation
(iii) Functional activities in a developmental sequence
(iv) Balance activities
(v) Frenkel's exercises
(vi) Use of lead weights
(vii) Gait retraining

POLYNEUROPATHY

Disorder of peripheral nerve function which results generally in a flaccid paresis and/or a peripheral sensory disturbance. Symptoms are frequently symmetrically distributed.

Common causes

A broad classification is:
1. Metabolic — e.g. diabetes mellitus
                                porphyria
2. Dietetic — e.g. vitamin B deficiencies
                            alcoholism
3. Miscellaneous — e.g. Guillain-Barré
4. Infective — e.g. leprosy
5. Chemical — e.g. side effects of drugs — Ionazid
                            heavy metals — lead, arsenic
6. Secondary — associated with: collagen diseases
                                                            sarcoidosis
                                                            carcinoma
7. Hereditary — peroneal muscular dystrophy

Pathology

Axonal degeneration and/or segmental demyelination

Signs and symptoms

1. Motor — weakness, paresis, initially distally, but progressing proximally
2. Sensory — numbness, paraesthesia of glove and stocking distribution, often accompanied by an unpleasant burning sensation and considerable pain

Medical treatment
1. Directed towards alleviation or cure of basic cause
2. Assisted ventilation if required

Guillain-Barré syndrome
Frequently preceded by a 'flu' like illness. Onset is acute, and deterioration may be rapid, progressing to include not only peripheral muscles, but also those of respiration. Sensory involvement tends to be less marked. Steroids may be given to arrest or reverse the course of the disease.

Assessment of all polyneuropathies
1. Respiration
   (i) Rate of respiration
   (ii) Chest expansion
   (iii) Vital capacity
2. Motor power
3. Sensation
   (i) Cutaneous
   (ii) Proprioceptive
4. Joint range
5. Function

Principles of physiotherapy
1. Maintain airway and adequate ventilation by:
   (i) Breathing exercises
   (ii) Postural drainage, vibration, assisted coughing
   (iii) Assisted ventilation – see page 85
2. Maintain joint range and muscle length by:
   (i) Passive movements
   (ii) Positioning and splinting
3. Strengthen affected muscles by:
   (i) Neuromuscular facilitation techniques
   (ii) Progressive resistance exercises
   (iii) Equilibrium and righting reactions
   (iv) Free active exercises
   (v) Springs and pulleys
   (vi) Suspension therapy
   (vii) Afferent cutaneous stimuli
   (viii) Hydrotherapy
4. Increase sensory awareness by:
   (i) Cutaneous stimulation
   (ii) Use of alternative sensory pathways – e.g. vision
5. Re-educate function by:
   (i) Activities of daily living
   (ii) Choice and use of aids

FACIAL PALSY (Bell's palsy)

Acute unilateral peripheral lesion of the seventh cranial nerve. Frequently it results from pressure caused by inflammation of the nerve within the facial canal.

Common causes
1. Idiopathic
2. Herpes Zoster of geniculate ganglion (Ramsay Hunt Syndrome)
3. Middle ear conditions
   (i) Infection
   (ii) Complications of surgery

Signs and symptoms
On affected side:
1. Loss of facial expression
2. Loss of eye closure
3. Loss of ability to purse lips or retract angle of mouth
4. Ballooning of cheek on mastication and respiration
5. Loss of taste of anterior two-thirds of tongue if lesion occurs in proximal part of facial canal

Medical treatment
1. Steroids to minimize swelling in facial canal
2. Analgesics for pain relief

Principles of physiotherapy
Re-education of facial muscles by:
1. Active exercises
2. Neuromuscular facilitation techniques
3. Splinting
4. Care of cornea
Note: (i) Eighty per cent of all idiopathic facial palsy recovers within four weeks

PERIPHERAL NERVE INJURIES

Types of injury

Neuropraxia
1. Loss of conduction without degeneration
2. Nerve conduction possible below lesion
3. Sensory modalities frequently less affected than motor, and autonomic least of all
Prognosis: Good – Recovery usual within six weeks

Axonotmesis
1. Disruption of axon, but nerve sheath intact
2. Wallerian degeneration is followed by axons regrowing to own end organs
Prognosis: Good – Time scale depends on site of lesion

Neurotmesis
1. Disruption of axon and nerve sheath
2. Surgery required to approximate nerve sheaths and enable growing axon to reach correct end organ

Prognosis: Variable — Functional recovery dependent on axons reaching correct end organs

In neuropraxia and neurotmesis classical signs of nerve degeneration are seen — clinically and electrically

Wallerian degeneration
1. Nerve degenerates proximally to nearest node of Ranvier and distally throughout whole length
2. Debris cleared by macrophagic activity
   Process takes up to 21 days to complete and is a preparation for regeneration

Nerve regeneration
1. Regenerating axons send out many branches, one of which becomes myelinated and continues to grow down the neural tube
2. Growth rate approximately 1 mm per day
   It occurs unevenly throughout the regeneration period, being initially faster
   Factors influencing rate:
   (i) Age of patient
       faster in younger age group
   (ii) Site of lesion
        faster when lesion is more proximal to spinal cord
   (iii) Nature of lesion
         faster following spontaneous regeneration than following nerve suture

Signs and symptoms

Motor
1. Flaccid paralysis
2. Muscle wasting
3. Loss of tone and deep reflexes
4. Shortening of unopposed muscle groups

Sensory
1. Cutaneous loss
2. Proprioceptive loss

Autonomic
  1. Temperature change
  2. Loss of sweating
  3. Trophic disturbances
      (i) Loss of hair
      (ii) Delayed healing of wounds
      (iii) Brittleness of nails

Assessment

Motor
  1. Manual muscle testing
  2. Electrical testing
      (i) Nerve conduction testing up to 21 days
      (ii) Strength duration curve after 21 days

Sensory
  1. Localization of touch
  2. Proprioception
  3. Two point discrimination
  4. Temperature

Autonomic
Sweat test – may not be routinely used

Range of joint movement

Principles of physiotherapy
1. Maintain or increase circulation by
   (i) General activity of limb
   (ii) Massage
   (iii) Elevation
2. Maintain or restore full range of movement by
   (i) Passive movements
   (ii) Neuromuscular facilitation techniques
   (iii) Free active movement
   (iv) Use of splints
      a. Rest splints
      b. Serial splints
3. Increase strength in unaffected muscles and affected muscles by
   (i) Neuromuscular facilitation techniques
   (ii) Balance and equilibrium reactions
   (iii) Free active exercise
   (iv) Progressive resistance exercise
   (v) Springs and pulleys
   (vi) Suspension
   (vii) Hydrotherapy
4. Re-educate sensation by:
   (i) Heightening sensory awareness
   (ii) Retraining stereognosis
5. Promote function
   by:
   (i) Use of trick movements
   (ii) Use of lively splints
   (iii) Games and activities

Nerve suture
Necessary to approximate nerve ends following neurotmesis may be:
1. PRIMARY — sutured up to six hours following trauma, if wound clean
2. SECONDARY — sutured around three weeks after trauma. The nerve ends are previously secured to prevent retraction

Post operative regime

Time	Immobilization	Principles of physiotherapy
1–3 weeks	Immobilized in plaster with nerve in shortened position. Limb may be elevated	1. Maintain circulation 2. Encourage activity in unaffected joints
3–8 weeks	Gradual mobilization avoiding stretch on nerve	as above plus: 3. Increase range of movement within prescribed limits
		4. Increase strength in unaffected muscles
8 weeks onwards	Full mobilization	See 'Principles of Physiotherapy' page 162

Individual nerve lesions

Axillary nerve — C5 and 6
Motor Supply:
1. Deltoid
2. Teres minor
Sensory supply:
Skin over deltoid muscle
Deformity:
Flattening of contour of shoulder
Functional disability:
Loss of ability to abduct and elevate arm
Common causes:
1. Dislocation of shoulder
2. Fracture of upper end of humerus

Radial nerve — C5, 6, 7, 8, T1
Motor supply
1. Triceps
2. Anconeus
3. Brachioradialis
4. Extensor carpi radialis longus
   via posterior interosseous nerve:
5. Extensor carpi radialis brevis
6. Supinator
7. All long extensors of fingers
8. Extensor carpi ulnaris
9. Abductor pollicis longus
10. Extensors of thumb
Sensory supply via posterior cutaneous nerve of arm
1. Posterior aspect of upper arm
   via lower lateral cutaneous nerve of arm
2. Lateral aspect of upper arm
   via posterior cutaneous nerve of forearm
3. Posterior aspect of forearm
   via terminal radial nerve:
4. Dorsum of radial side of hand including thumb.
Deformity
1. Wrist drop
2. Wasting of extensor muscles of forearm
Functional disability
1. Loss of synergic action of wrist extensors leads to weak flexor
   grip
2. Inability to place objects on flat surface
Common causes
1. Pressure in axilla
   (i) Crutches
   (ii) Arm hanging over back of chair
2. Fracture shaft of humerus
3. Trauma at elbow joint

Median nerve — C6, 7, 8, T1
Motor supply
1. Pronator teres
2. Flexor carpi radialis
3. Palmaris longus
4. Flexor digitorum superficialis
5. Flexor digitorum profundus
6. Flexor pollicis longus
7. Pronator quadratus
8. Abductor pollicis brevis
9. Opponens pollicis
10. Flexor pollicis brevis
11. 1st and 2nd lumbricals

Sensory supply
1. Palmar aspect of thumb, index, middle and half ring fingers and corresponding palm
2. Dorsum of terminal phalanx of index, middle and half ring fingers

Deformity
1. Monkey hand — thumb lies in same plane as palm
2. Wasting of thenar eminence
3. Indicating gesture — loss of flexion of index finger and partial loss of flexion of middle finger

Functional disability
1. Loss of precision grip
2. Loss of kinaesthetic sense of radial side of hand

Common causes
1. Laceration at wrist
2. Compression in carpal tunnel
3. Trauma at elbow

Ulnar nerve — C8, T1
Motor supply
1. Flexor carpi ulnaris
2. Medial half flexor digitorum profundus
3. Palmaris brevis
4. Hypothenar muscles
5. Medial two lumbricals
6. Palmar and dorsal interossei
7. Adductor pollicis
8. Flexor pollicis brevis

Sensory supply
1. Palmar aspect of little finger and half ring finger and corresponding palm
2. Dorsal aspect of little finger and half ring finger

Deformity
1. Claw hand – hyperextension of 4th and 5th metacarpo-phalangeal joints and flexion of interphalangeal joints
2. Drift of little finger into abduction
3. Wasting of hypothenar eminence and interossei.

Functional disability
1. Loss of power grip
2. Loss of precision movements of fingers

Common causes
1. Laceration at wrist
2. Trauma at medial epicondyle of elbow.

Common peroneal nerve – L4, 5, S1, 2

Motor supply
1. Biceps – short head
2. Tibialis anterior
3. Extensor digitorum longus
4. Extensor hallucis longus
5. Extensor digitorum brevis via Musculotaneous nerve
6. Peroneus brevis
7. Peroneus longus

Sensory supply
1. Antero-lateral surface of lower leg
2. Web of first and second toes.

Deformity
1. Loss of anterior muscle bulk giving sharply defined tibial edge
2. Foot drop

Functional disability
1. High stepping gait
2. Equinovarus position of foot.

Common causes: Pressure at neck of fibula by
1. Tight plaster of paris
2. Trauma at time of fracture

FURTHER READING

Adams, G. F. (1974) *Cerebrovascular Disability and the Ageing Brain.* Edinburgh: Churchill Livingstone.

Atkinson, H. W. (1974) *Neurology for Physiotherapists.* ed. Cash, J. E. Ch. 1–6. London: Faber & Faber.

Bannister, R. (1969) *Brain's Clinical Neurology.* London: Oxford University Press.

Bobath, B. (1969) The Treatment of neuromuscular disorders by improving pattern of co-ordination. *Physiotherapy,* **55**, 1, 18.

Bobath, B. (1970) *Adult Hemiplegia, Evaluation and Treatment.* London: Heinemann.

Burns, A. (1975) *Loss of Higher Neurological Function.* Adelaide: Lutherian Publishing House.

Chusid, J. G. & McDonald, J. J. (1973) *Correlative Neuro-Anatomy & Functional Neurology.* Oxford: Lange Medical Publications.

Blackwell Scientific Publications.

Ciba Foundation Symposia (1975) *Outcome of Severe Damage to the Central Nervous System.* Amsterdam: Elsevier.

Goff, B. (1972) The application of recent advances in neurophysiology to Miss M. Rood's concept of neuromuscular facilitation. *Physiotherapy,* **58**, 12, 409.

Haines, J. (1967) Survey of recent developments in cold therapy. *Physiotherapy,* **537**, 222.

Hollis, M. (1977) *Practical Exercise Therapy.* Oxford: Blackwell Scientific Publications.

Hooper, Reginald (1969) *Patterns of Acute Head Injury.* London: Arnold.

Jennett, W. B. (1977) *An Introduction to Neurosurgery.* (London: Heinemann.

Knott, M. & Voss, D. E. (1968) *Proprioceptive Neuromuscular Facilitation (Hocher).* London: Balliere.

Lane, R. E. J. (1969) Physiotherapy in the treatment of balance problems. *Physiotherapy,* **55**, 10, 415.

McLeod, J., French, E. B. & Munro, J. F. (1974) *Introduction to Clinical Examination.* Edinburgh: Churchill Livingstone.

Medical Research Council, (1972) *Aids to the Investigation of Peripheral Nerve Injuries.* London: H.M.S.O.

Payton, O. D., Hirst, S., Newton, R. A. (1977) *Scientific Bases for Neurophysiologic Approaches to Therapeutic Exercise.* Philadelphia: F. A. Davis Co.

Peterkin, H. W. (1969) The neuromuscular system and the re-education of movement. *Physiotherapy,* **55**, 4, 145.

Seddan, Hubert (1975) *Surgical Disorders of the Peripheral Nerves.* Edinburgh: Churchill Livingstone.

Stoddard, J. C. (1975) *Intensive Therapy.* Oxford: Blackwell Scientific Publications.

Todd, J. M. (1974) Physiotherapy in early stages of hemiplegia. *Physiotherapy,* **60**, 11, 336.

Waddington, P. J. (1975) *Chest, Heart and Vascular Disorders for Physiotherapists,* ed. Cash, J. E. Ch. 3–4. London: Faber & Faber.

Walshe, F. (1973) *Diseases of the Nervous System.* Edinburgh: Churchill Livingstone.

Williams, Moyra (1970) *Brain Damage and the Mind.* Harmondsworth: Penguin.

Geriatric physiotherapy

DEFINITION

The branch of physiotherapy dealing with the remedial, social and preventative aspects of the elderly disabled and disadvantaged

COMMON GERIATRIC PROBLEMS

Cardiovascular disease
1. Myocardial infarction
2. Myocardial ischaemia (angina pectoris)
3. Intermittent claudication (angina cruris)
4. Gangrene. Chronic leg ulcers
5. Hypertension
6. Postural hypotension
7. Heart valve disorders
8. Varicose veins
9. Varicose ulcers
10. Deep venous thrombosis
11. Congestive cardiac failure

Central nervous system disease
1. Cerebral atherosclerosis
2. Carotid region syndromes
   (i) Transient ischaemic attacks (TIA)
   (ii) Thrombosis
   (iii) Embolism
   (iv) Haemorrhage
3. Vertebro-basilar region syndromes
   (i) TIA
   (ii) Thrombosis
   (iii) Embolism
   (iv) Haemorrhage
   (v) Drop attacks
   (vi) Cervical spondylosis
4. Parkinsonism

Alimentary disease
1. Hiatus hernia
2. Diverticulosis
3. Peptic ulcer
4. Malabsorbtion
5. Carcinoma — oesophagus, stomach, colon, rectum

Common alimentary symptoms
1. Constipation
2. Dysphagia

Dietary disorders (not as common as generally believed)
1. Scurvy (Vitamin C deficiency)
2. Pellagra (Vitamin B complex deficiency)
3. Vitamin B_{12} deficiency
4. Vitamin D deficiency
5. Folate deficiency
6. Iron deficiency
7. Obesity — very common
8. Protein deficiency

Diabetes
1. Mainly adult onset
2. Ulcers
3. Neuropathy

Anaemias
1. Iron deficiency
2. Megaloblastic
3. Of chronic disease
   (i) Chronic renal failure (uraemic)
   (ii) Rheumatoid
   (iii) Bowel disease
   (iv) Infected ulcers and pressure sores
   (v) Tuberculosis

Infections
1. Pneumonias
2. Urinary tract infections
3. Tuberculosis

Disorders of homeostasis
1. Electrolyte imbalance
   (i) Hypokalaemia (often from use of diuretics)
   (ii) Hyponatraemia
2. Dehydration
3. Hypothermia
4. Hyperthermia

Eye disease
1. Glaucoma
2. Cataracts
3. Diabetic retinopathy
4. Optic lesions following stroke

Hearing disorder
1. Nerve deafness
2. Bone conduction deafness

Musculoskeletal disorders
1. Osteoarthritis
2. Rheumatoid arthritis
3. Rare collagen diseases (e.g. SLE, dermatomyositis)
4. Pagets disease
5. Osteoporosis
6. Osteomalacia
7. Tumours
8. Causes of back pain
    (i) Osteoporosis
    (ii) Osteomalacia
    (iii) Osteoarthrosis
    (iv) Paget's disease
    (v) Prolapsed disc
    (vi) Tumour

Common fractures
1. Femoral neck: subcapital and transcervical
2. Femoral: intertrochanteric and subtrochanteric
3. Neck of humerus
4. Colles

Causes of falls
1. Cerebral
    (i) drop attacks
    (ii) TIA
    (iii) Epilepsy
    (iv) 'Faints'
2. Cardiovascular
    (i) Postural hypotension
    (ii) Stokes-Adams attacks

Mental confusions and dementia
1. Dementia
   (i) Primary
   (ii) Secondary (to cerebral arteriosclerosis, tumour etc.)
2. Confusion (delirium)
   (i) Acute
   (ii) Subacute

Causes
   a. Infections e.g. Pneumonias, UTI
   b. Retention of urine
   c. Cerebral Hypoxia — Cardiac failure
                        — Severe anaemia
                        — Respiratory failure
   d. Carcinomatosis
   e. Cerebral ischaemia
   f. Myxoedema
   g. Nutritional — Pellagra
                  — Scurvy
                  — Vitamin B_{12} and folate deficiency
   h. Social — Bereavement
             — General upheaval
   i. Drugs — Barbiturates
            — L-dopa
            — Digitalis
            — Alcohol
   j. Organic cerebral lesions — Tumour
                               — Epilepsy
                               — Parkinsonism
                               — Sub-dural haematoma

Urinary incontinence
1. Stress incontinence
2. Unstable bladder
3. Senile vaginitis
4. Chronic bacteruria
5. Carcinoma of bladder
6. Prostatic hypertrophy
7. Neurogenic bladder

Faecal incontinence
1. Constipation — overflow incontinence
2. Neurogenic
3. Abuse of laxatives
4. Symptomatic
   (i) Side effects of drugs
   (ii) Diabetes
   (iii) Diverticular disease
   (iv) Carcinoma
   (v) Rectal prolapse

Pressure sores
1. Arteriosclerotic
2. Terminal
3. 'Normal' — caused by:
   (i)   Direct pressure
   (ii) Shearing forces
   (iii) Folding of skin

PARKINSON'S DISEASE

Aetiology
1. Idiopathic
2. Toxic — Manganese, Copper, Carbon monoxide
3. Drugs — Phenothiazines, Butyrophenones, Methyl dopa
4. Metabolic — Wilson's disease
5. Repeated trauma
6. Post encephalitic
7. Arteriosclerotic

Signs and symptoms
1. Tremor — Pill rolling
2. Rigidity — Leadpipe and cogwheel
3. Bradykinesia
4. Hypokinesia
5. Defective postural reflexes
6. Lack of facial expression — Parkinsonian facies
7. Shuffling gait — Festinant
8. Difficulty with starting and stopping walking
9. Autonomic symptoms
   (i)   Excessive salivation
   (ii) Flushing
   (iii) 'Feels hot'
10. Stretch reflexes — May be increased

Treatment
1. Drug therapy
   (i) L dopa
   (ii) L dopa plus carbidopa
   (iii) Anticholinergics
   (iv) Amantadine
   (v) Penicillamine in Wilson's disease and toxic Parkinsonism
2. Surgery — Stereotactic surgery to basal ganglia
3. Physiotherapy
   (i) Assess for:
      a. Contractures
      b. Altered muscle tone
      c. Reduced joint range
   (ii) Treatment:
      a. Passive movements
      b. Active exercises
      c. Relaxation exercises
      d. Reduce contractures
   (iii) Schedule:
      a. Passive movements. Slow, rhythmical and full range
      b. Active exercises:
         Assisted, free or resisted
         Sling exercises
         Manually resisted exercises
         Spring exercises
      c. Relaxation exercises:
         Pendular and rhythmical
         Sling exercises
      d. Reduce contractures:
         Strengthen weakened muscles
         Passive movements
         Active movements

Other neurological diseases see p. 151

MANAGEMENT IN HOSPITAL OF THE MULTI-PATHOLOGY GERIATRIC PATIENT

Team approach
All members assess on admission and discuss

Team members
1. Physiotherapist
2. Doctor
3. Nurse
4. Occupational Therapist
5. Speech Therapist
6. Social Worker

Ward rounds and conferences

Continual reassessment and collation of information so that each team member is aware of progress and the aims and mode of treatment being given by each other member.

Encourage independence

The patient should contribute to his treatment by:
1. Dressing
2. Managing the toilet
3. Making own bed
4. Taking own tablets
5. Walking whenever possible
6. Performing taught exercises on own
7. Performing small tasks – buttering bread etc.
8. Talking to staff – important if speech problem

Discharge

Discuss with patient – assess attitude
Discuss with involved relatives – assess attitude
Home visit essential if patient residually disabled – even if relative or help at home

Home visit

Take patient to home during the day with at least two team members
Aim:
1. Assess ability to cope in own home
2. Decide if any equipment may be needed to help
3. Assess services required to support at home

RESETTLEMENT AT HOME

Facilities available to support at home:

1. Warden Service
   Help get patient out of bed, washed and dressed. In evening put them back to bed
2. District Nurse
   Injections, dressing, catheter care
3. Meals on Wheels
   Hot lunch, usually twice a week
4. Home help
   Clean House, do washing, buy food, prepare meals, sometimes collect pension. Usually provided three times a week
5. Bath Attendants
   Under supervision of District Nurse. Gives either normal or blanket bath
6. Night Attendants
   Nurses who sit with patient perhaps two nights a week to relieve relatives
7. Health Visitor
   Makes frequent visits to check patient is managing
   Refers if necessary
8. Social Worker
   Becomes involved if problems develop outside the scope of the Health Team
9. Laundry Service
   Washing of linen and clothes of incontinent patients
10. Chiropodist
    Visits patients unable to get to clinics

Other facilities to aid support at home

1. *Day centre:*
   Run by Social Services to provide a day out plus lunch
2. *Day hospitals:*
   Run by National Health Service with close attachment to a hospital. Designed for continuation of previous in-patient care/patients referred for rehabilitation.
   Reasons for attendance:
   (i)   Medical
   (ii)   Nursing
   (iii) Physiotherapy
   (iv)   Occupational therapy
   (v)   Speech therapy
   (vi)   Social (for relative relief) for
   (vii) Maintenance of severely disabled
3. *Old age pensioner clubs:*
   Run by various charity groups, churches etc.
   e.g. Darby and Joan Clubs, Over 60's.
4. *Aids for use in the home*
   (i) *Walking aids*
        a.   Frame: Gutter frame, Rollator, Reciprocal
        b.   Stick
        c.   Quadrapod
        d.   Crutches
   (ii) *Wheelchairs*
        Many varieties according to needs. Motorized/non-motorized
   (iii) *Bed aids*
        a.   Hospital bed (adjustable height)
        b.   Rubber mattress and cover
        c.   Bed cradle
        d.   Rubber ring
        e.   Overhead monkey pole
        f.   Rope ladder

   (iv) *Bath aids*
- a.   Bath seat
- b.   Bath board
- c.   Non slip mat
- d.   Hoist
- e.   Hand grips

   (v) *Toilet aids*
- a.   Raised toilet seats
- b.   Hand grips on wall
- c.   Frame around toilet
- d.   Commodes
- e.   Urinals
- f.   Bedpans
- g.   Incontinence pads
- h.   Incontinence sheets

5. *Adaptations to home* (by Social Services if necessary)
   - (i)   Ramps for wheelchair access
   - (ii)   Extra hand rails on stairs
   - (iii)   Raise height of chairs
   - (iv)   Widen doors
   - (v)   Alter kitchen for wheelchair existence
   - (vi)   Special worktops in kitchen

PRINCIPLES OF TREATMENT

Deal with the complete person
Their mental, social and physical needs
Don't ignore problems other than physiotherapy ones
Example

A 75 year old obese diabetic woman with bronchopneumonia, mild congestive cardiac failure and osteoarthritic knees. Patient lives alone in a small terraced house with outside WC, and upstairs bedroom, sole means of heating coal fires. Her daughter normally visits once per week. Until four weeks ago, managed well with help from a stick and neighbours who did little shopping. Fell in back yard four weeks ago. On ground for half an hour. Found by neighbour who helped her inside and called GP. No injury found but now unable to get around. Therefore sleeps on settee and uses commode emptied by daughter daily. Two days ago, developed cough and pyrexia. Admitted to hospital.

Initial investigations
1. Chest X-ray
2. Urine analysis and culture
3. Blood urea and electrolytes
4. Full blood count
5. Blood sugar
6. Culture and sensitivity of sputum
7. ECG

Treatment ordered
1. Broad spectrum antibiotic
2. Physiotherapy
3. Mild diuretics

Later diet specified for obesity and diabetes, and analgesia given for painful joints.

Physiotherapy treatment
Initially:
1. Postural drainage, taking into account the mild congestive cardiac failure
2. Breathing exercises
   (i)   Diaphragmmatic
   (ii) Lateral costal
   (iii) Apical
3. Gentle clapping and shaking
4. Deep cough to remove secretions
5. Leg exercises
   (i)   Ankle dorsi and plantarflexion
   (ii) Static quads drill
   (iii) Knee flexion and extension (active)
   (iv) Static gluteal exercises

Treatment as above initially twice a day within tolerance of patient

Assessment and progression
Once Broncho-pneumonia has resolved continue breathing exercises to
ensure maintenance of a clear chest
1. Assess joint range passively and actively of lower limbs
2. Assess muscle power of lower limbs

Progression
Once patient is allowed out of bed more active and intensive treatment
can be started.

Treatment
1. Infra-red to knees
2. Static Quads drill
3. Active knee flexion and extension
4. Straight leg raising
5. Active arm exercises
6. Standing practise

Progression

Treatment
1. Continue Infra-red to knees
2. Resisted knee flexion and extension
3. Resisted straight leg raising
4. Walking in parallel bars

Progression

Treatment
1. Check patient able to get in and out of bed
2. Check able to move around in bed
3. Check ability to get up off floor
4. Practise doing stairs
5. Practise walking on uneven surfaces
6. Walking with frame

Progression

Treatment
Walking with stick

Occupational therapy

Activities of daily living
1. Dressing
2. Cooking
3. Washing
These must all be assessed and able to perform them unaided prior
to discussion of discharge.

Physiotherapy assessment
1. Patient can now manage stairs with handrail
2. She can get in and out of bed and on and off commode placed by side of bed
3. Walking independently with the aid of a stick
4. Cannot get up off the floor without assistance because of pain and stiffness in knees

Discharge
1. Patient very anxious to return home
2. Daughter prepared to continue support
3. Case conference discusses patient's progresses and with reports from all members of the team it is decided to do a home visit

Home visit
Members of team
1. Physiotherapist
2. Occupational therapist
3. Social worker
4. Home help organizer if possible to assess if home help will be required

To assess possible problems. Can she:
1. Manage the stairs?
2. Walk to the outside toilet?
3. Make up coal fire in living room?
4. Prepare meals in her own kitchen?

Results
1. Stairs will need second handrail as stairs are very steep and patient very anxious to sleep upstairs
2. She can manage to get to outside toilet
3. Very difficult to make up fires — suggested to daughter that a gas fire be installed, with which she agrees and will make necessary arrangements.
4. Patient will be able to cook a simple meal

On discharge
Day hospital — twice a week to maintain a check on her diabetes, dieting and to make sure patient continues to make progress
Home help — once a week to do heavy washing, collect pension and to do shopping. Also to do heavy cleaning of house

LIVING ACCOMMODATION AVAILABLE FOR GERIATRICS OTHER THAN THEIR OWN HOMES
Long stay wards in NHS Hospitals

Old people's homes
1. Part three accommodation
2. Run by the Social Services

Private nursing homes
1. Some run by charity organizations
2. Some run by church organizations
3. Some run by industrial organizations for retired employees

Warden controlled flats — Council flats with a resident warden

Alm's Houses

Purpose built Old Age Pensioner flats

ORGANIZATIONS FOR GERIATRICS

Help the Aged. 8–10 Denman Street, London W1A 2AP.
Age Concern and British Geriatrics Society. 60, Pitcairn Road, Mitcham, Surrey CR4 3LL.
Central Council for the Disabled. 34, Eccleston Square, London SW1V 1PE.
British Association for Services to the Elderly. Home 1, Office 12, University House, Well Lane, South Manchester M20 8LR.
Disabled Living Foundation. 346, Kensington High Street, London W14 8NS.
National Corporation for the Care of Old People. Nuffield Lodge, Regents Park, London NW1.

FURTHER READING

Anderson, F. (1976) Preventative aspects of geriatric medicine. *Physiotherapy*, **62**, 5, 146.

Anderson, W. F. (1971) *Practical Management of the Elderly*. Oxford: Blackwell Scientific Publications.

Anderson, W. F. & Judge, T. G. eds. (1974) *Geriatric Medicine*. London: Academic Press.

Brocklehurst, J. C. (1970) *The Geriatric Day Hospital*. London: King Edward's Hospital Fund.

Brocklehurst J. C. (1976) The day hospital. *Physiotherapy*, **62**, 5, 148.

Brocklehurst, J. C. & Hanley, T. (1976) *Geriatric Medicine for Students*. Edinburgh: Churchill Livingstone.

Caird, F. I. (1976) Diagnosis in old People, *Physiotherapy*, **62**, 6, 178.

Cash, J. E. (1974) *Neurology for Physiotherapists*. London: Faber & Faber.

Goble, J. E. & Nichols P. J. R. (1971) *Rehabilitation of the Severely Disabled*. London: Butterworths.

Hawker, M. (1974) *Geriatrics for Physiotherapists and Allied Professions*. London: Faber & Faber.

Hodhuson, H. M. (1975) *An Outline of Geriatrics*. London: Academic Press.

Isaacs, B. (1965) *Introduction to Geriatrics*. London: Baillere.

Isaacs, B. (1976) The place of a stroke unit in geriatric medicine, *Physiotherapy*, **62**, 5, 152.

Judge, T. G. (1976) Nutrition in the elderly, *Physiotherapy*, **62**, 6, 179.

Kennedy, B. F. (1976) The stroke unit: A physiotherapists view, *Physiotherapy*, **62**, 5, 154.

Kennedy, R. D. (1976) Teamwork in geriatric medicine, *Physiotherapy*, **62**, 5, 158.

Mandelstam, D. A. (1976) Incontinence, *Physiotherapy*, **62**, 6, 182.

Mary Marlborough Lodge (Eds.) (1974) *Equipment for the Disabled*. 3rd edn. Nos 1–10. London: National Fund for Research into Crippling Diseases.

Marston, P. D. (1976) Day hospitals: A physiotherapists view, *Physiotherapy*, **62**, 5, 151.

Robinson, R. A. (1976) Mental Illness in the elderly, *Physiotherapy*, **62**, 5, 155.

Skin disorders and burns

SKIN DISEASES

Acne vulgaris

Pathology
1. Increased activity of sebaceous glands
2. Raised sebum production leads to blocked gland ducts
3. Infection occurs
4. Pustules form
5. Area round pustules inflamed
6. Common sites, neck, face, upper back
7. Cause, changes in endocrine activity, diet
8. Occurs at puberty

Principles of physiotherapy
1. Obtain desquamation of skin
2. Increase vascularity
3. Reduce number micro-organisms
4. Improve general health and hygiene

Methods
1. Teach normal skin care and hygiene
2. UVR dosage $E_2{}^o$
3. Scheme exercises to improve posture and movement
4. Cosmetic preparations for greasy skins
5. Advice on diet

Psoriasis

Pathology
1. Dilatation of capillaries in dermis
2. Oedema of epidermis, leading to:
3. Increased activity of stratum germinosum
4. New cells form horny scales
5. Removal scales reveals pin-point bleeding
6. Sexes equally affected
7. Cause, endocrine metabolic, familial
8. Associated with rheumatoid arthritis

Principles of physiotherapy
In sub-acute/chronic stage
1. Remove horny scales
2. Improve general health
3. Allay psychological fears

Methods
1. Coal tar bath/paste
2. UVR
   (i) General suberythemal dose
   (ii) Local $E_2{}^o$ to remove tough scales
3. Soothing ointment if skin sore

BOILS AND CARBUNCLES

Pathology
1. Infection of hair follicle
2. Pus formation under skin and subcutaneous tissues
3. Pus discharges to surface
4. Cause, friction, constitutional disorder

Principles of physiotherapy
Post drainage
1. Encourage drainage of pus
2. Improve general health
3. Advice on prevention of reoccurrence
Methods
1. SWD
2. UVR $-$ E_4 to pus area
3. Medical $-$ antibiotics, diet.

GRAVITATIONAL ULCER

Pathology
1. Venous stasis, due to varicosities, thrombus, gravity
2. Poor tissue circulation
3. Area indurated
4. High protein content in oedema
5. Skin damaged by minor trauma
6. Ulcers form and become infected
7. Oedema may reduce joint movements
8. Site $-$ near tibial malleolus
9. Examine with magnifying glass
10. Trace ulcer for records

Appearance of ulcer
Floor $-$ red, may contain pus/slough
Lips $-$ hard, red, non-healing
Base around ulcer $-$ erythematous/pigmented

Principles of physiotherapy
1. Improve venous and lymphatic drainage
2. Combat infection
3. Mobilize foot and ankle joints
4. Strengthen muscles of lower leg (muscle pump action)
5. Encourage WB activities in patient
6. Encourage weight reducing programme

Methods
1. Elevation
2. Pressure bandaging
3. Bisgaard massage techniques
4. Faradism – under – pressure
5. UVR
6. Ice cube massage
7. US
8. Passive mobilization
9. Active and resisted exercises
10. Increase daily walking/cycling
11. Advice on care ulcer and life-style

PRESSURE SORES

Pathology
1. Caused by ischaemia of superficial tissues, due to body weight
2. Shearing forces between tissue planes
3. Examine sore using illuminated magnifying glass
4. Tracings of sore initially and at intervals

Types of sore
1. Infected:
   (i) Dry, hard, black slough
   (ii) Thin, stringy, soft pus
2. Indolent: uninfected, clean, non-healing
3. Clean healing

Principles of physiotherapy
Local
1. Remove slough and pus
2. Reduce infection
3. Increase tissue resistance to mechanical trauma
4. Improve circulation
5. Increase rate healing

General
1. Build up general body resistance
2. Prevent further sores
3. Strengthen postural muscles
4. Teach transfers

Methods

Local
1. UVR
    (i) To remove slough dosage $E_4^o \times 10$
    (ii) To indolent sore dose E_3^o
    (iii) To healing wound E_2^o + abiotic filter
    (iv) To base area E_1^o
2. Ice cube massage to sore, dosage 5 min
3. 2 hourly turning

General
1. Postural exercises
2. Transfers
3. General UVR E_1^o
4. Diet and antibiotics

BURNS

Classification
1. Superficial partial thickness
2. Deep partial thickness
3. Full thickness

Effects
1. Shock – loss proteinous tissue fluid
2. Anaemia
3. Infection
4. Kidney damage
5. Cardiac failure

Principles of physiotherapy

Medical
1. Prevent circulatory failure
2. Control infection
3. Improve general health
4. Facilitate healing-graft

Physiotherapy
1. Prevent contractures
2. Remove oedema
3. Maintain joint range
4. Maintain muscle bulk
5. Improve circulation
6. Prevent respiratory infection
7. Reassure patient

Skin grafts

Types
1. Full thickness
2. Partial thickness
3. Free grafts
   (i) Split skin
   (ii) Full thickness
4. Flap grafts
   (i) Tubular
   (ii) Fixed base

Special points re: skin grafts
1. Avoid stretching and massage techniques
2. Care in exercise not to cause oedema/haemorrhage under graft
3. Do not disturb skin grafts
4. No direct heat
5. Care using splinting
6. Avoid infecting graft

FURTHER READING

Cash J. E. (1976) *Textbook of Medical Conditions for Physiotherapists.* London: Faber & Faber.

Index